Prevent Cancer Now

Also by Dr. Michael Colgan:

Electrodermal Responses
The Training Index
The Power Program
Your Personal Vitamin Profile

Prevent Cancer Now

Second Edition

Your Guide to Self-Protection

Michael Colgan, Ph.D.

C.I.Publications
San Diego, 1992

For information contact C.I. Publishing
531 Encinitas Blvd., Encinitas, CA 92024

This book is NOT intended for the treatment of disease, not as a substitute for medical treatment, nor as an alternative to medical advice. It is a review of scientific evidence presented for information purposes, to increase public knowledge of developments in the field of cancer prevention.

SECOND EDITION

Library of Congress Cataloging in Publication Data

Colgan, Michael, 1939 -

Prevent Cancer Now

Bibliography: p.
Includes index.
1. Cancer prevention. 2. Health.
I. Title.

Library of Congress Catalog Card Number 89-81363

ISBN 0-9624840-2-4 (cloth)

ISBN 0-9624840-3-6 (pbk)

Printed in the United States of America

Contents

	Foreword	vii
	Introduction	ix
	Acknowledgments	xi
1.	The War Against Cancer	1
2.	The Future is Prevention	8
3.	No Smoke Without Cancer	14
4.	Excess Alcohol Promotes Cancer	17
5.	Overweight Causes Cancer	19
6.	Low Calories Prevent Cancer	27
7.	Low Fat Diet Prevents Cancer	30
8.	High Fiber Prevents Cancer	40
9.	Vegetables Prevent Cancer	44
10.	Refined Foods Promote Cancer	49
11.	Vitamins and Minerals Prevent Cancer	53
12.	Antioxidents Prevent Cancer	63
13.	Immunity Against Cancer	74
14.	Essential Fatty Acids Prevent Cancer	79
15.	Don't Drink The Water	83
16.	Food Pollution Causes Cancer	88
17.	Cancer On The Job	98
18.	Keep Cancer Out Of The House	103
19.	Ultra-Violet Causes Cancer	107

21. Exercise Prevents Cancer 115
22. Screening Helps 118
23. The Anti-Cancer Lifestyle 121

Tables

Table 1: Cancer Risk Factors 10
Table 2: The Relative Risks for Death by Cancer 13
Table 3: Popular Diets that Fail to Provide Proper Nutrition 23
Table 4: Ranking of Fats and Cholesterol in 30 High Protein Foods 33
Table 5: Fat per Serving 36
Table 6: Fat Content of High Fat Snacks 39
Table 7: Fat Content of Low Fat Snacks 39
Table 8: Fiber "10" 43
Table 9: Anti-Carcinogenic Produce 48
Table 10: Top Twenty Grains and Legumes 52
Table 11: Nutrient Intake of Sample of 37,785 U S Citizens 56
Table 12: Multi-Vitamin/Mineral Basic Formula 61
Table 13: Daily Amounts of Antioxidants used to Prevent Animal Cancers 78
Table 14: Essential Fatty Acids in Oils 83
Table 15: How to Minimize Pesticide Residues in Produce 92
Table 16: Occupational Exposure to Carcinogenic Metals 102
Table 17: The Cancer Prevention Lifestyle 124

Foreword

Cancer.

The word itself causes a strong reaction in most of us. It evokes images of a slow painful death. Our food, our water, our homes, even our air seems to cause cancer and nothing seems to cure it.

Traditional medicine offers us surgery, chemotherapy, and/or radiation as treatments, all of which may cause cancer themselves. Yet even taking this risk, the cancer patient has less than a 50% chance of effecting a remission or stopping the spread of cancer through their body. Non-traditional medical approaches to dealing with cancer also focus on curing the cancer victim. Their effective cure rate is, at best, no better than traditional medicine has to offer.

Processes such as the macrobiotic diet, various approaches to visualization, the Gerson diet, as well as different psychotherapies provide some hope but, quite frankly, not much. It boils down to this; once you've got cancer, it takes a tremendous amount of work, energy, faith and luck to get rid of it. The odds aren't good. Yet there has to be some way of dealing with this life-threatening problem.

Into this dilemma steps Dr Michael Colgan, a world renowned scientist. Dr Colgan has previously focused on helping athletes maximize their performance as well as helping the general public optimize their health through nutrition and supplementation. In this book, he turns his attention towards developing a common sense approach to the problem of cancer. An approach that, while not easy, is effective. An approach that anyone can understand and implement.

Using the most up to date research from the world over and employing the same vigorous, systematic, impeccable scientific approach he is noted for, Dr Colgan offers us a way out — a way to Prevent Cancer Now.

David Cornsweet, Ph.D.

Introduction

I am a scientist not a physician. My research is on nutrition, exercise and lifestyle interventions, and their effects on bodily function. My expertise is in analyzing the results of scientific research and assessing the implications of those results for human life.

I am not trained in dispensing medical advice. That is the exclusive function of your physician. The information in this book is not an alternative to medical advice, nor a substitute for medical treatment. It is an analysis of evidence that certain nutrition, exercise, and lifestyle practices can prevent cancer.

I urge you to consult the scientific and medical references given herein, to decide for yourself the merits of my analysis. You should also pursue other references, as this is only a small book, covering only a tiny fraction of the research. I have done my best to ensure that it covers the most important work, but new studies appear every day. Dr David Cramer, for example, at Harvard Medical School, has just reported that some women do not metabolize galactose properly. Galactose is a sugar found in dairy products, that is toxic to some people. Failure to metabolize it increase the risk of ovarian cancer.

You see, cancer is a complex problem. We are only just learning to prevent it. So some of the practices described herein, such as the taking of large amounts of certain nutrients, are still highly experimental. If you choose to pursue them, you do so upon your own responsibility. No one should take large doses of vitamins or minerals without consulting a physician trained in nutrition. Some diseases can be adversely affected by nutrients, and nutrients can adversely affect some prescribed medications.

Because of such complications, your approach to nutrition and lifestyle protection against cancer, must be careful and informed. Nevertheless, it is possible to prevent this grim disease, and **you**, by your own actions, are the only one who can do it. I wish you well.

Michael Colgan, Ph.D.

San Diego, CA

November, 1989

Acknowledgments

In 1982 I watched a wonderful woman, Bo Modell, die helplessly of cancer. Since that time I have made cancer the model of my research into degenerative processes. I have been helped along this road by so many good people, it is impossible to name them all. Let my thanks to a few apply equally to everyone.

Dr Linus Pauling gave me the encouragement and insight to realize how nutrients can inhibit all degeneration. Dr. Jonas Salk, showed me how **host resistance** is the key to all disease. Dr Michael Brines, my friend and mentor at Rockefeller University, guided me to all the crucial papers on prevention. Dermatologist, Dr Zein Obagi, taught me how human skin is truly the mirror of human health. Plastic Surgeon, Dr Dennis Nigro, shaped my awareness of the physics of human structure. Dr Walter Mertz convinced me, that man is indeed but a fragile enlivenment of a handful of the elements of Earth.

For this manuscript, thanks to Dawn Mariani, whose meticulous word-processing and incisive commentary pushed me through the writing and re-writing, to the last reluctant comma.

Thanks most of all to my fellow scientist and companion in research, my wife, my love, Lesley Colgan, who encouraged and cajoled and helped beyond measure to spread this good, so generously given me, before you, so that the more may benefit.

To Megan,
My lady in the making

Chapter 1

The War Against Cancer

Cancer is grim. Once you develop it the chance of a **cure** is less than 50/50. You, by your own actions, have a far better chance of **preventing** this disease. You can eliminate 90% of the threat of cancer from your life. To the extent that you do so, you eliminate the second largest cause of death.

First you have to know the facts. In 1971, President Nixon declared a knockdown, dragout "war on cancer". Billions of tax dollars were allocated and the people rejoiced. The crab would be beaten at last. Every year since then the US National Cancer Institute has claimed enormous progress. As we enter the 1990's, it has become obvious that many of these claims are false.

If you cannot believe that the official war on cancer has been a failure, and you have to learn to protect yourself, then examine the medical and scientific studies from which this book is drawn. Throughout, I have documented every conclusion with references to impeccable research. The Colgan Institute is an independent research and educational organization. We have no axe to grind against health authorities. We are simply presenting the scientific facts in a form that is easily understandable, and therefore of greatest help to everyone.

The sad truth is, cancer patients die in America today, at a faster rate than they did in the "prewar" days of the fifties and sixties. On May 8th 1986, in the *New England Journal of Medicine*, cancer specialists Dr John Bailor of the Harvard School of Public Health and Dr Eileen Smith of the University of Iowa published meticulous figures showing that cancer survival has not improved at all (1). On the contrary, from 1950, to the latest figures available for the 1980's, the cancer death rate has actually **increased**.

Bailor's research echoed the views of many cancer researchers and other medical insiders. Among them, throughout the 1980's, writers for the Colgan Institute have published numerous critical articles in its journal *Nutrition & Fitness* (2). The message from all these scientists, was that the National Cancer Institute was failing in its task to reduce cancer. Meanwhile, the public is constantly reassured by health authorities that all is well and getting better.

The storm of scientific protest finally alerted government. Representative Ted Weiss (D-NY) demanded an investigation by the General Accounting Office, the watchdog division of Congress. The GAO findings, released in April 1987, concluded that, "*the extent of improvement in survival for specific cancers is often not as great as that reported*" (3).

So all is not well. We are losing the war against cancer. In 1962 cancer deaths in America totalled 280,000. In 1982 they totalled 435,000. That's a 56% increase. But, of course, the population has also grown. The increase in the number of people at risk has to be taken into account. When you adjust for our larger population, cancer deaths have still increased by a whopping 25%.

The National Cancer Institute objects to these figures, saying that the U.S. population is also getting older. So more people are in the age groups at greater risk for cancer. Therefore, says NCI, you would expect an increase in cancer.

The aging of America **does** put more of the population at greater cancer risk. But Bailor at Harvard took this into account (1). With all possible biases accounted for, the cancer death rate is still increasing. Nine more patients in every 100 cases die of cancer today than in 1950. We are definitely losing the war.

Its A Bloody Rout

Breast cancer, the third leading cause of cancer death in America, is one area where the National Cancer Institute claims great success. Vincent De Vita, Director of NCI, claims a significant reduction in breast cancer mortality. I wish he was right. He bases this claim on the increased number of patients who survive five years after diagnosis, a condition often called a **cure** among looser-lipped denizens of the cancer industry.

In the 1950's, about 60% of women diagnosed

with breast cancer survived five years. Now the figure is 75%. But that is not the 15% improvement in treatment that De Vita would have us believe. George Silverman, Director of the General Accounting Office, points out that breast cancer is now being **detected** earlier. It is usually a slow-growing cancer that can take 10-15 years to become obvious, and often 20 years to kill.

With more cases of breast cancer being detected at an earlier stage of development, then it follows that more will still be alive five years later, because the disease has to progress for a longer period before it becomes terminal. So De Vita's **improvement in treatment** has little to do with advances in treatment, and mostly to do with counting more cases earlier. After analyzing all the data, the GAO report concluded there was a "*slight improvement in survival*" (3).

There's that word "survival" again. You see how easily even the GAO gets bamboozled by the term **five year survival.** The real issue is, are more women dying of breast cancer or not? Unfortunately, more women are.

Let us be generous to NCI, and leave out all the women over 50, who NCI claims bias the figures, because they are at greater risk. Meticulous research,using NCI's own figures for cancer deaths, shows that, during the 1980's, **the breast cancer death rate in young women has increased** (3,4).

I didn't examine breast cancer because it was **the** bad case. All the leading cancers are bad cases. The number one cause of cancer death is lung cancer. And lung cancer in America is increasing astronomically. Scientists have various abstruse theories to explain this increase in illness in a land with more doctors and medicine than anywhere else on Earth, but it doesn't take a genius to see the truth. No one wants to accept it, but we have fouled our own nest. Every day our air, water, food and environment become more and more polluted.

On 12 April 1989, the Environmental Protection Agency reported that the level of toxic wastes released daily into our land, air, and water is *"far higher than we thought"*. They first obtained the alarming data from the national inventory of toxic wastes, taken in 1987. The report, just now completed, shows a total of 22.5 billion pounds of pollutants released in that year alone. Almost 10 billion pounds were poured into rivers, streams and lakes. Another 2.7 billion pounds fouled our air. Most of the rest was dumped into pits to foul our land.

Don't believe that federal health authorities can protect you. They are almost powerless. The Environmental Protection Agency is so inneffective, that on May 26, 1989, John Van de Camp, State Attorney General of California, together with a group of organizations concerned with our declining environment, filed a lawsuit against the EPA, charging that they had failed in their appointed task to protect the nation against carcinogens.

So it should be no surprise that lung cancer is increasing, or that the five-year survival rate for lung cancer remains a miniscule 10%, about the same as it was in 1960. Remember, that's not a cure. When we look at the correct measure, that is, the death rate from lung cancer, then NCI's **Cancer Statistics Update** shows that a higher proportion of lung cancer patients are dying than in 1960. **We are not only losing the war against cancer, its a bloody rout.**

It's time the public was told in plain language, that the cancer picture is grim. The National Cancer Institute agrees that one American in every three will get cancer (5). For 1989 alone, the Surgeon General's report predicts over 900,000 new cases (6). Yet the chance of a cure is slimmer than ever.

Compiled from official figures, Figure 1 shows that the cancer death rate in America has increased steadily since 1960. All the efforts and billions of dollars in former President Nixon's "*war against cancer*" have not even put a dip in the graph.

Don't let these facts depress you. You can provide your body with powerful weapons against cancer. These weapons are all derived from recent advances in science. But you don't have to be a genius to understand them. Nor do you have to buy expensive medical technology or services. They are simple, straightforward, and convenient for daily use by everyone.

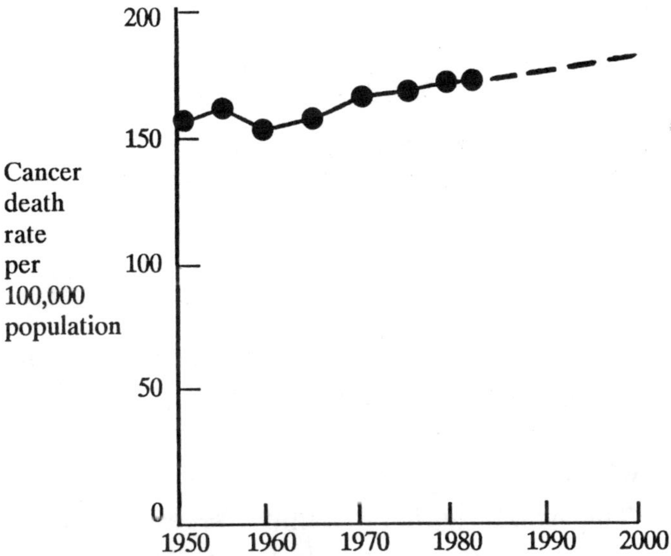

Source: Adapted from Bailor, *New England Journal of Medicine*, 8 May 1986, p. 1226.
*Projection by the Colgan Institute bascd on NCI figures to 1989.

Figure 1. Mortality from cancer in the United States Population (age adjusted to US population of 1980 to allow for general aging of population). If this allowance is not made, increase in cancer mortality is considerably worse than shown here.

Chapter 2

The Future is Prevention

The answer to all major cancers lies not in surgery, drugs or radiation therapy. These procedures, though essential for treatment, have such a high failure rate, that we have to find another way.

The answer lies in prevention. Yet even now, in 1990, less than 1% of cancer dollars is spent on prevention. Over 99% is spent on treatment, much of it ineffective, all of it wildly expensive.

Medical science is not focussed on prevention of cancer because it is almost impossible to get money for it. Unlike a tumor to cut out, you can't see prevention. It earns no fat fees, sells no drugs, confers no status, hones no surgical skills, provides no immediate medical gratification at all. No person or agency can convincingly claim the credit for prevention. Few therefore, are motivated to try.

Prevention happens slowly, by education, by the dissemination of information that you can use yourself. Prevention happens when you realize that no physician, hospital, or government agency can protect you against cancer. You have to learn to protect yourself. Self protection is what this book is about.

Remember, you do not die of old age. You die of disease. You do not become a feeble, medically dependent geriatric because of the passage of time, you become that way because of degenerative processes that have been growing in your body for many years. Cancer is predominantly a degenerative disease. Most cancers grow silently inside you for decades, before being discovered. They do not occur at all in healthy bodies.

Before you can develop cancer, your body has to lose or damage many of its defense mechanisms. In the healthy person, these mechanisms destroy cancer cells every day. Esteemed British scientist and physician, Sir Peter Medewar, was fond of saying in lectures, that the average person gets cancer a million times in his life. The healthy body destroys every one of these budding cancers long before they become established.

Cancer is the second biggest cause of death and infirmity in Western Society. It is also the most feared, the most macabre. Yet the risk factors for 99% of all cancers are known. They are listed in Table 1. Over 90% of these risks are avoidable. To the extent that you avoid them, you avoid the disease.

I am sure the evidence presented in these pages will convince you that you can do it.

Table 1. Cancer Risk Factors
1. Smoking
2. Exposure to smokers
3. Excess alcohol
4. Overweight
5. Excess calories
6. High fat diet
7. Low fiber diet
8. Low vegetable and fruit diet
9. High use of processed foods
10. Vitamin and mineral deficiencies
11. Diet low in antioxidants
12. Essential fatty acids deficiencies
13. Known cancer risk industries
14. Pollutants in faucet water
15. Pollutants in foods
16. Environmental pollutants
17. Sunlight
18. Sedentary life style
19. Radon gas and radiation
20. Failure to have cancer check-ups
21. Medications and medical treatment

Sources: American Cancer Society,
U. S. National Cancer Institute, Colgan Institute

Cancer Prevention Strategy

So many things are shown to cause cancer today, from the chlorine in drinking water to Alar on our apples, that many people just give up trying to fight it. Uninformed media, focused on circulation profits rather than human health, have us running scared at negligible risks of cancer, while failing to inform us of the real risks.

To the average person, pesticides seem a far greater cancer risk than being overweight. In fact, the reverse is true. Cancer risk from overweight is many times that of all the pesticides on our food put together (5a, 5b).

The Colgan Institute gets numerous requests from individuals and organizations to apportion risk for different carcinogens. Although this is a difficult task, and cannot be exact, we have used figures from the National Cancer Institute, The American Cancer Society, from cancer expert Professor Bruce Ames of the University of California (Berkeley), from British cancer experts Drs Richard Doll and Richard Peto and from our own fifteen years of computer records of all major studies.

Our analysis is summarized in Table 2. It indicates the way you should worry about cancer. Causes you cannot avoid are listed separately.

The table makes it clear that a smoker who worries more about environmental pollution is being idiotic. A mother who stuffs her children with high fat chips and dips, yet refuses to buy apples because they may have traces of Alar, is sadly ignorant of reality. And a person who eats the average American diet, but plasters on the sunscreen to prevent skin cancer, just doesn't know where the big risks lie.

I want you to know the big risks. Successful prevention of cancer is partly a numbers game. I might bet against the 2% risk of sunlight, but never against the 33% risk of smoking. For successful prevention of cancer, first kick out the big ones.

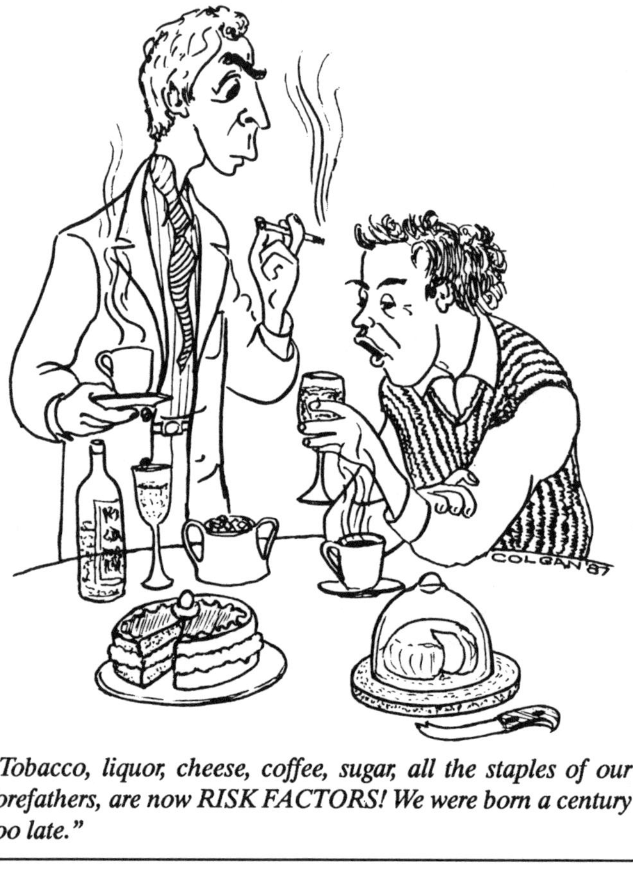

"Tobacco, liquor, cheese, coffee, sugar, all the staples of our forefathers, are now RISK FACTORS! We were born a century too late."

Table 2: The Relative Risks for Death By Cancer

Avoidable Causes of Cancer	% of US Cancer Deaths
Smoking (including chewing tobacco)	33%
Eating Excesses	25%
Nutrient deficits	15%
Environmental pollution (including pollutants in foods, air and water)	5%
Sunlight	2%
Prescription Drugs	2%
Illicit drugs and excess alcohol	1%
Radon Gas	1%
Radiation	1%

Unavoidable Causes of Cancer	% of US Cancer Deaths
Viruses and Infectious Agents	7%
Genetic defects	2%

Source: The Colgan Institute, Encinitas, CA

Chapter 3

No Smoke Without Cancer

Smoking heads the list in Table 1 as the biggest single risk factor for cancer. Back in 1979, in his **Report on Health Promotion and Disease Prevention**, the then Surgeon General stressed that smoking causes over 80% of all lung cancers, and up to half of all bladder cancers (10).

You have only a 10% chance of surviving lung cancer. And that includes lung cancer from second-hand smoke. In 1987, the then Surgeon General, Dr Everett Koop, presented compelling reports from the American Lung Institute, that inhaling smokers' air increases cancer risk.

In one study, Dr Pelayo Correa and colleagues, at the Louisiana State University Medical Center in New Orleans, examined 1,338 lung cancer patients in Louisiana and compared them with controls. They found that non-smokers married to heavy smokers had an increased risk of lung cancer. Even adult children of mothers who smoked showed an increased risk (10a). Studies in other Westernized countries, including

Japan, have had similar findings (10 b, 10 c). Secondhand smoke is definitely carcinogenic.

You risk more than just lung cancer from tobacco smoke. The National Cancer Institute also indicts smoking as a major cause of pancreas cancer, kidney cancer, mouth cancer, throat cancer, and uterine cancer (5).

NCI also released a statement on March 17, 1989 citing new evidence. These studies confirm that smoking also causes cervical cancer. Cigars, pipes, snuff and chewing tobacco are indicted also, especially for mouth and throat cancers.

Smoking is a prime example of gradually creating a degenerative process in your body. In lung cancer, smoking over a number of years progressively damages all cells within the lung, and progressively weakens the immune defense systems that protect delicate lung tissues. Finally the defense systems fail to eliminate a cell that has become malignant, and it starts to grow a cancer.

Don't believe the insidious hypocrisy of tobacco supporters, that good nutrition and regular exercise can protect you against the ravages of smoking. Yul Brynner kept his body in superb condition. He ate the best nutrition and exercised vigorously. His one problem was smoking. He smoked all his adult life and gave it up only when he learned he had developed lung cancer. Too late. Despite the best treatment in the world, he died miserably of cancer at the height of his career.

It's never too late to stop smoking **before** you get cancer. One year after you quit, lung cancer risk is reduced by a whopping 50%! In ten years, it is likely that your lungs can recover completely.

Don't smoke! And don't let others puff their smoke about you. If you are a smoker now, you cannot be serious about longevity. It is worth paying all you have, to stay in a substance abuse clinic until you stop smoking. If you don't, then every other step you take to protect your health will come to naught.

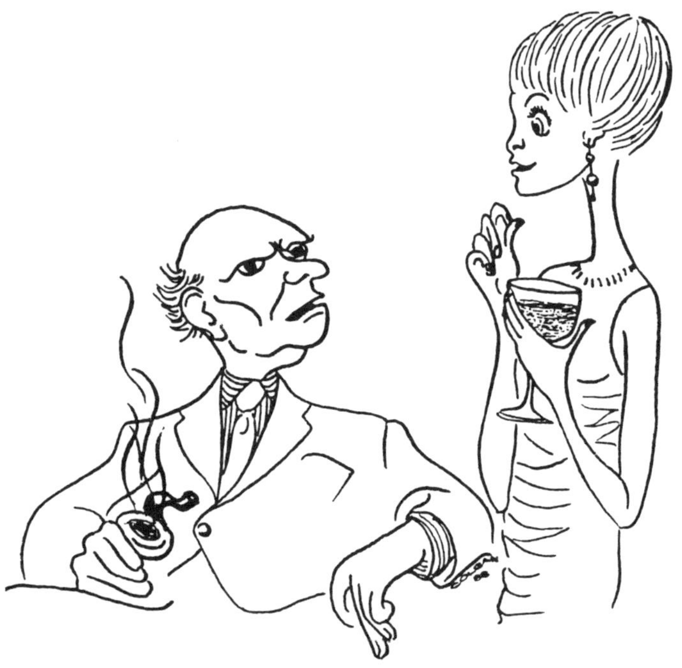

"Got to keep smoking, dear. If I don't have my morning cough, your grandmother has me doing all sorts of chores."

Chapter 4

Excess Alcohol Promotes Cancer

Studies of the National Cancer Institute link alcohol use with cancers of the mouth, throat, oesophagus, and liver (5). In their prestigious report, *Diet, Nutrition and Cancer*, The U. S. National Research Council also connected excessive beer drinking with colorectal cancer (26). It's worse if you are a smoker. The report concluded that smoking and alcohol add together to increase the risk of cancer of the mouth, throat and lungs.

The connection between alcohol and cancer is more subtle than it is with smoking. Alcohol causes cancer in fewer people, and does not seem to be directly causative. The National Research Council suggests that it may not be the alcohol itself. Other non-alcoholic components of beer, wines and liquor may be responsible.

Over 1,000 chemicals are added to alcoholic beverages and, up to the present, the alcohol industry has successfully resisted all attempts even to tell the public what the chemicals are. It is a sad commentary on American society, that we insist on non-carcinogenic cookies being labelled down to the last innocuous ingredient, while carcinogenic alcohol mixtures continue to feed us hundreds of toxins blind.

At least we know that it is excess use of alcohol that causes cancer. But how much is excess? Good estimates indicate that one American in every five drinks too much (7). That's over fifty million of us! Confirmed alcoholics total 17 million (8). With that level of alcohol consumption, it's contribution to the cancer load must be enormous.

We don't know exactly how much alcohol causes cancer. But it's a good bet that the level of intake that causes degenerative disease is the signal to stop drinking. A survey of relevant studies by the Colgan Institute agrees with the conclusion reached by a similar survey by the Harvard Medical School. More than one-and-a-half ounces of alcohol per day results in slow degeneration of the liver, which in turn increases risks of both cardiovascular disease and cancer (9).

A regular size drink contains approximately half an ounce of alcohol. So the upper limit, if you want to prevent cancer, seems to be three beers OR three glasses of wine OR three singles of liquor. To stay on the safe side, keep it at a maximum of two drinks a day.

Chapter 5

Overweight Causes Cancer

Overweight really means overfat. For millions of years of evolution, Mother Nature programmed the human organism to store fat against times when food was scarce. Most of us have a very efficient fat storage system, which gets even more efficient as we age.

Some researchers suggest that the evolutionary reason for this is that aging humans are less able to catch and gather food. So the ones who survived by natural selection, were those who developed fat storage mechanisms that increased their fat storage function with age. They are our ancestors.

Now we no longer need that function, because food is never scarce. So we get fat, and more and more easily fat, as we age. Permitting yourself to become fat, is permitting a general degenerative process to occur that is linked to many diseases. Premature aging and early death are almost inevitable in the overweight. And cancer is very likely.

In 1959, the American Cancer Society mounted a massive 20-year study of over one million Americans in 25 different states. At the end of the study in 1980, results showed unequivocally that overweight causes cancer. Men who are 40% or more overweight have higher rates of cancer of the prostate, colon and rectum. Women who are more than 40% overweight have higher rates of cancer of the breast, uterus, ovaries and gall bladder (11). Staying slim is not just pandering to vanity. For healthy longevity it is essential.

Slim is easy to say, but hard to do, with our inherited tendencies to store fat, forever shaping us into waddling blimps. As a nation, America is fatter today than it was 20 years ago. Obese is 25% or more above ideal weight. Now, almost one woman in every three, and one man in every six is technically obese (12). It's a standing joke that America has enough excess fat stored to feed the whole of starving Africa -- and that most of our overweight would gladly pay to donate it.

How did we get in this state? For more than a decade now we have seen an explosion of health clubs, miracle diets, appetite suppressants, "lite" foods, weight loss clubs and, Lord save us from ourselves, the ultimate indignity of liposuction. Why can't we beat the flab?

The plain fact is, most diets make you fatter. Yes, **fatter**. Read on. The evidence will convince you. American dieting tends to be the crash variety. Starve today for a svelte Saturday night. Chew celery sticks for a month to fit that new outfit. Pig out at Christmas, then diet all spring to get lean and tan for the beaching days of summer.

If you reduce your calories to the point of hunger pangs and weakness, your body does lose fat quickly, but only temporarily. Such rapid dieting, promoted by most popular diets, increases production and biological activity of a fat storage enzyme called lipoprotein lipase. When you go off the diet, this enzyme continues to be overactive. It collects the fat you eat and deposits every molecule again with such efficiency, that your bodyfat is soon higher than it was before you started (13). As a direct result of dieting, you have **increased** your bodyfat.

Dieting also slows your resting metabolic rate, so it becomes harder for your body to use excess calories for energy. New studies by Dr Diane Elliot and colleagues, at Oregon Health Sciences University in Portland, show that this reduced metabolic rate can persist for two months following a diet of the same duration (14).

During that post-diet period, the reduced metabolic rate alone can put back most of the fat you lost, even if you eat lightly. Combining reduced metabolism with the overactive fat storage enzyme, and a stringent diet of two months duration, can result in you being five pounds heavier than ever four months later. Do this once a year, and in 10 years you will be 50 lbs fatter. No wonder America's obsession with intermittant dieting is making us the fattest nation on Earth.

Dangerous Diets

Popular diet books are used for much of America's dieting. Almost all of them rely on reducing calories to the point where the diet becomes too low in vitamins, minerals and other nutrients. So you not only put on more fat, you endanger your health with nutrient deficiencies as well. A study by Dr Paul La Chance and Michelle Fisher at Rutgers University in New Jersey shows that all the diets listed in Table 3 are deficient in one or more essential nutrients (15).

The study found that some very popular diets, such as the Stillman Diet, the Richard Simmons Diet, the Beverly Hills Diet and the Scarsdale Diet were seriously deficient in vitamins and minerals.

The Beverly Hills Diet, for example, provided only half of the Recommended Dietary Allowance of niacin and riboflavin, less than two-thirds of the RDA of thiamin and pyridoxine, and virtually no vitamin B12. It also provided only one-third of the RDA of calcium and one-quarter of the RDA of zinc. Such a deficient intake is an invitation to disease.

Most of the diets were also too low in fiber. As you will see in Chapter 8, the National Cancer Institute now recommends 25-35 grams of fiber per day as a cancer preventative. **None** of the diets in the La Chance study provided this amount. For most of them, intake was less than 12 grams, with the Stillman, Atkins and Richard Simmons diets providing less than 5 grams.

Table 3: Popular Diets That Fail to Provide Proper Nutrition

Diet	Worst Deficiencies
Atkins	Vits. B1, B6, Folic Acid, Iron Calcium, Magnesium, Fiber
Beverly Hills	Vits. B1, B2, B3, B6, Calcium Phosphorous, Iron ,Zinc, Fiber
Carbohydrate Cravers	Vits. B6, B12, Folic Acid, Iron, Zinc, Fiber
California	Vits. B6, B12, Fiber
F Plan	Vit. B12, Calcium, Fiber
I Love America	Vits B1, B6, Folic Acid,Iron Magnesium, Zinc,Fiber
I Love New York	Vit. B6, Fiber
Pritikin	Vit. B12, Zinc, Fiber
Richard Simmons	Vits. A, B1, B2, B6, B12, Folic Acid, Calcium, Iron Magnesium, Zinc, Fiber
Scarsdale	Vits. B1, B2, B6, B12, Folic Acid, Calcium, Magnesium, Iron, Zinc, Fiber
Stillman	Vits. A, C, B1, B6, Folic Acid, Calcium, Magnesium, Iron, Fiber

Source: Adapted from Fisher and LaChance, 1985 (15).

Medical Diets

What about the new fad for those expensive *medically supervised diets?* They are certainly better than self dieting. These programs, such as Optifast and Medifast, rely on liquid meal replacements, and make sure that the diet is complete in nutrients, at least to the standard of the Recommended Dietary Allowances (RDAs).

But they still face the same problem of too much fat loss too fast, which activates lipoprotein lipase and slows metabolism. As soon as you stop the diet, you immediately start to blimp up. The Colgan Institute followed thirteen people who lost bodyfat on this type of program. Eight of the subjects regained most of the lost fat within 12-18 months. Five were successful in remaining slim, but none of these was very fat to begin with.

A larger study confirms our findings. In 1988, *The American Journal of Public Health* reported on 200 people who lost an average of 84% of their excess weight on these medically supervised diets. Within three years after the diet, they had regained 60-80% of the bulge (16).

The purveyors of these supervised programs do advise lifelong maintenance procedures to keep off the fat, but for most people the cost is prohibitive. The plain fact is that most do not continue. So if you rely on periodic diets to lose weight, medically supervised or not, you are probably doomed to be fat. And every pound of excess multiplies cancer risk.

Sensible Fat Loss

It is not difficult to control bodyfat, if you accept that it is a lifelong business, and you realize that the American food supply is stacked against you. Here are 10 lifetime rules that we have used successfully since 1974 at the Colgan Institute. Some people who started with us way back then have kept the fat off now for 15 years.

1. Never crash diet and never fast.

2. Lose bodyfat slowly: MAXIMUM loss permitted is one pound per week.

3. Reduce fat intake to 25% of calories or less. This is explained in the next section.

4. Avoid all fad diets. Don't buy diet books. Don't enroll in weight loss clubs or meal replacement programs.

5. Avoid sugars. Simple sugars, including honey, raw sugar and all fruit juices, cause insulin bursts that disrupt insulin metabolism and promote fat deposition.

6. Eat complex carbohydrates. Whole grains, legumes and vegetables reduce fat deposition by a variety of mechanisms.

7. Eat only sufficient calories. Learn to leave plates unfinished. The starving Africans your mother told you about will never know. If you must pig out save it for "occasions".

8. Maintain adequate chromium status. A recent US Dept of Agriculture study shows that Americans eat an average of less than 50 micrograms

of chromium a day (17). Long-term balance studies show that a daily intake of 200-290 micrograms is required to maintain chromium status (18). Without adequate chromium, a degenerative condition gradually develops called insulin resistance. Dr L Felig of Yale University has shown that insulin resistance slows the metabolic rate, thereby increasing deposits of excess calories as bodyfat (19). One 200 microgram capsule of chromium picolinate is an ample and safe supplement to maintain chromium status.

9. Regulate insulin production. Some of the above rules help to do this. In addition, eat at regular hours, eat a high fiber diet and include omega-3 fatty acids (fish oils) in the diet. Dr Leonard Storlien at the Garvin Institute of Medical Research in New South Wales, Australia, has shown that omega-3 fatty acids prevent insulin resistance (20). At least two meals per week of the cold-water fish, salmon, trout, sardines or mackerel will provide ample fish oils.

10. Exercise in the mornings. Morning workouts raise metabolic rate for some hours afterwards, thereby burning more calories throughout the day (21). Earlybird exercise also burns a higher proportion of bodyfat as fuel than does exercise later in the day.

Stick to these simple rules for lifelong lower bodyfat and reduced risk of cancer.

Chapter 6

Low Calories Prevent Cancer

When you have beaten the bogey of excess bodyfat, you might consider becoming super slim. Studies now indicate that maintaining a condition of very low bodyfat may not only prevent cancer, but also extend life by other mechanisms. Fifty years ago, Dr Clive McCay at Cornell University extended the lifespan of rats by more than 50%, by lifelong severe restriction of their caloric intake. The rats developed far fewer cancers than non-restricted rats (22). Since then Dr Maurice Ross has used the same technique to **double** rat lifespan (23). That is equivalent to extending human lifespan to two hundred years.

Most of us would not accept radical restriction of calories lifelong. Fortunately that is not necessary. Dr Benjamin Berg of Columbia University has reduced rates of cancer in rats and extended their lifespans with restriction of calories by only 33%.

Renowned gerontologist Dr Roy Walford and his colleagues at the University of California Medical School have done some of the best research on underfeeding. In a recent and representative study, they restricted the caloric intake of mice, until their bodyfat remained at a low level. Results showed that these very slim mice were healthier all round than their fatter litter mates. They developed far fewer cancers, remained sleek and active lifelong, and lived 10-20% longer than the controls (24).

In another excellent study, Walford and his co-workers found that one in every two of fully fed mice ultimately developed cancer. In the food restricted mice, only 13% developed cancer, that is one in eight. (24a) Remember, the National Cancer Institute reports that one in every three Americans will get cancer. (5) Undereating alone might well cut the human cancer rate in half.

In reducing rates of specific cancers, the under-feeding studies score even better. Breast cancer in some laboratory strains of female rats occurs in at least every second animal. In a study by Drs M. Ross and G. Bras, reported in the *Journal of the National Cancer Institute*, caloric restriction reduced the rate of this cancer to **zero** (24b).

There are two aspects of these studies that make them entirely different from the human dieting that goes on in America. First, the caloric restriction was regular and absolute. There was no way the animals could cheat or overeat at parties, weddings, funerals and gargantuan blow outs. So there was no yo-yoing of bodyfat, up and down, which is the usual human pattern with its attendant disruption to hormonal and metabolic functions.

Second, and even more important, these studies restricted calories, but all of them made sure that subjects received adequate supplies of vitamins, minerals and other essential food factors. As we discussed in Chapter 5, most reduction diets are woefully inadequate in nutrients. The secret is regular undereating without undernourishment. You cannot avoid cancer and achieve longevity unless you have adequate nutrition.

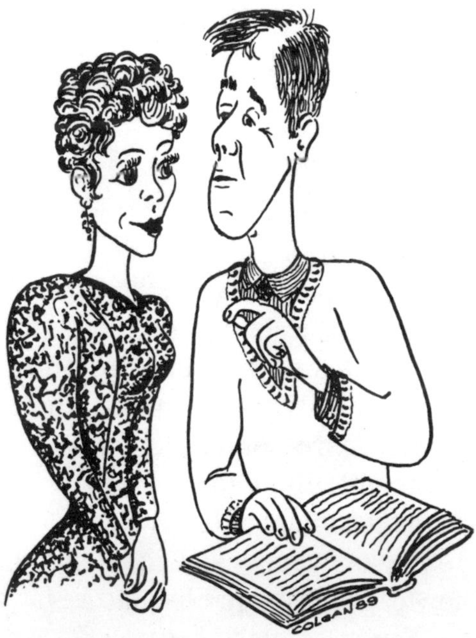

"We can make a fortune with a diet book that teaches people to eat wood - high fiber, low calories, low fat, low salt, low sugar - and look how tall and slim trees get."

Chapter 7

Low Fat Diet Prevents Cancer

The American population still eats a diet that is 42% fat. Yet all major US health authorities now recommend keeping fat intake below 30% of total calories. Because of the degradation of the American food supply, that's about as easy as opening a can of beans - with your lips.

In October, 1987, the New York Times surveyed the diets of 1,870 people. Over half the respondents claimed they had cut right down on fats and cholesterol in their diets. Yet their responses to other questions showed regular meals of red meats, whole eggs, fast foods, ice cream and other high fat foods. These people may have the intention to cut down, but lack the knowledge of fat content of foods that will enable them to do it. To prevent cancer you had better acquire this simple knowledge. You don't have to **be** fat in order to risk cancer. You just have to **eat** fat.

We know that dietary fat is a direct cause of cancer from animal experiments. A typical study, by Dr AW Bull et al, injected rats with a known carcinogen that reliably causes cancer in experimental studies. Then they fed one group a high-fat diet, about the level of fat in the American diet. They fed the other group a low-fat diet, about the level of fat in the Japanese diet. The high-fat group developed twice as many tumors as the low-fat group (25).

In the 1980's, the National Research Council of the US National Academy of Sciences published strong evidence, mostly from animal experiments, linking dietary fat to cancer of the breast, colon, and prostate (26). Breast cancer provides the grimmest example. As we discussed earlier, there has been no improvement in the breast cancer death rate since 1960. Once you get it, your chance of a cure is less than the toss of a coin. With 150,000 new cases in 1989, it is certainly a cancer we should take every step to prevent. Kicking the fat habit is one big step.

Don't think I am overstating the case by relying on animal experiments. The human evidence is just as compelling. Dr J Silverman reported a study of 47 countries comparing fat intake and cancer incidence. The higher the fat in the diet, the higher the rate of breast cancer (27). Also, when women with low rates of breast cancer, such as the Japanese, move to the continental US, their breast cancer rate rises to the American level.

Lower That Fat!

Don't despair. With a few simple rules of thumb, you can lower your fat intake dramatically. First, become an avid label reader for all packaged and processed foods. Refuse to buy any food that does not give the fat content. Fat content is given by weight, so add a zero to get the approximate calories of fat. Then find the total calories per serving of the food, always given on the label. If the fat calories are more than a quarter of the total calories, leave it on the supermarket shelf.

Take plain vanilla ice-cream for example. Fat content is 8 grams per serving. Add a zero to get 80 fat calories. Total calories per serving is 160. Fat content is 80/160, that is 50%. Not an acceptable food for regular use if you want to prevent cancer.

Contrast ice cream with low-fat frozen yogurt, which today can be made to taste just as good as ice cream. Fat content is 2 grams per serving. Add a zero to get 20 fat calories. Total calories per serving is 110. Fat content is 20/110, that is 18%. Low-fat frozen yogurt is a good, low-fat food.

Many staple foods have no fat labelling, especially protein foods such as meat, fish, eggs, and cheese. A second rule of thumb to avoid the high fat varieties is - fish first. If you just can't stomach a high fish diet, then Table 4 gives the Top 10 and the OK 10 of common protein foods. It also gives the Worst 10, foods you should avoid if you want to prevent cancer.

Table 4: Ranking of Fats and Cholesterol in 30 High Protein Foods**

Top Ten Less Than 5% Fat	O. K. Ten 5% to 20% Fat	Worst Ten 30% to 60% Fat
Eat These		**Avoid These**
Cod	Shrimp*	Beefburger*
Sole	Tuna*	Pork Roast
Halibut	Chicken Breast	Bologna
Flounder	Duck Breast	Frankfurters
Lobster	Sardines	Beef Roast*
Crab	Herrings*	Bacon
Mussels	Salmon	Steak, T-Bone
Scallops	Lamb or Veal	Pork Sausage*
2% Cottage Cheese	Ricotta Cheese	Cheddar Cheese*
Turkey Breast	Eggs*	Cream Cheese*

** Fat Content by weight

* Over 100 mg cholesterol per 100 gm serving: Eggs have over 500 mg per 100 gms.

Source: Colgan Institute, Encinitas, CA

Label Gobbledegook

Don't be fooled by slick labelling, such as the big headlines on some packaged meat products that proclaim "*90% fat free*". Not bad, we are led to believe, only 10% fat. That's just advertising baloney on the bologna. The label figure states fat **by weight**, which is the legally allowed description. When you work out the percentage of fat calories, the story is just the opposite. Even the traditional low fat turkey can be rolling in fat. When the Colgan Institute analyzed a popular brand of turkey roll, it came out like this:

Turkey Roll:	
Water weight	70%
Fat weight	10%
Protein Weight	20%

The water has zero calories, the fat is 9 calories per gram and the protein is 4 calories per gram. So in an average 100 gram (3 1/2 oz) serving you get:

Water:	70 grams	=	0	calories
Fat:	10 grams	=	90	calories
Protein:	20 grams	=	80	calories
Total:		=	170	calories

The actual fat content of this supposed low-fat turkey roll is 90/170, a whopping 53%! That's a higher fat content than regular ice cream.

Don't be fooled by the words "Natural", "Wholegrain", "Lite", or "Lower Fat" either. Any copywriter worth his pencil can dodge round the laws governing use of words on labels. And beware those crafty graphics of wagon wheels, wooden butter churns, rich, dark piles of grains, friendly farmers' faces and down home goodness. Most of them came straight from Madison Avenue. The **contents** of the boxes may be anything but healthy.

Take the new Quaker cereal "**100% Natural**". The box looks great, all whole grain and raisins. But the ingredients label shows it has 5 grams of fat per serving. In contrast, Quaker's old standby **Puffed Wheat** has zero grams of fat per serving.

Shopping for Fat

Many people coming to the Colgan Institute complain that you can avoid fat only by eating foods that taste like sawdust, that you cannot get equivalents to normal food. Not so. Table 5 shows a typical shopping basket of cereal, bread, yogurt, crackers, snacks, cheeses, meat, dressing, candy and ice cream. On the smart side a day's fat intake from all these foods is only 16 grams. On the dumb, cancer promoting side it is 104 grams. The choice is yours.

Table 5: Fat per Serving

Item	Smart Choice	Fat (gms)	Dumb Choice	Fat (gms)
Cereal	Quaker Puffed Wheat	0	Quaker 100% Natural	5
Yogurt	Yoplait Light	0.5	Yoplait Custard Style	5
Bread	Wholewheat Breadsticks	1	Bran Muffins	8
Crackers	Ak Mak Crackers	2	Keebler Wheatables	6
Cheese	Lifetime Cheddar	3	Kraft Casino Cheddar	9
Cottage Cheese	Weight Watchers 1%	1	Skaggs Regular	5
Meat	Zacky Farms Turkey Roll	1	Oscar Meyer Bologna	8
Butter	Butter Buds	0	Regular Butter	11
Dressing	Tasti Italian	0	Lawry's Italian	9
Snacks	Mini Ricecakes	0	Butter Thins	6
Candy	Fibar Raspberry	3.5	Kudos Granola Bar	12
Ice Cream	Dryers Grand Light-Mocha	4	Hagen-Daz Mocha	20
Total Grams Fat	**Smart**	**16**	**Dumb**	**104**

Source: Colgan Institute, Encinitas, CA

Cut Out The Chips

Potato chips, corn chips, crackers, puffs, rinds, stix and bits all appear to be dry foods, therefore not high in fat. Wrong! Most dry crackers are so high in fat that major brands, such as Nabisco, don't dare put the fat content on the label, for fear of losing customers.

Companies that produce lower fat types of crackers do include a fat analysis, but even these are way above our cutoff of 25% fat calories. Hains Stoneground Wheat Cheese Crackers for example, are about 130 calories per serving with 3 grams protein, 17 grams carbohydrate and 6 grams fat. Our simple rule of thumb is to add a zero to the fat and compare it with total calories, that is 60/130. The crackers are over 40% fat, way past the healthy limit of 25%.

To work it out more accurately:

Protein:	3 grams = 12	calories
Carbohydrate:	17 grams = 68	calories
Fat:	6 grams = 54	calories
Total:	134	calories

Fat content is 54/134. That is, 40.2% fat.

Astute readers might object that I chose cheese crackers, and biased the deal because cheese is high in fat. Not so. These days the cheese flavor is only a fine film on the cracker surface. Most of the fat is inside. Take dry water crackers such as Pepperidge Farm Symphony Crackers. You can't get dryer than that.

Pepperidge Farm Symphony Crackers:

Protein:	1 gram	=	4	calories
Carbohydrate:	40 grams	=	40	calories
Fat:	3 grams	=	27	calories
Total:		=	71	calories

Fat content is 27/71, which is 38% fat.

Puffs and chips, stix and bits are much worse. Ruffles plain potato chips, for example, are:

Protein:	1 gram	=	4	calories
Carbohydrate:	15 grams	=	60	calories
Fat:	10 grams	=	90	calories
Total:		=	154	calories

Fat content is 90/154, which is 58% fat.

Table 6 gives the fat content of common brands of chips and other snacks you should avoid. You should also avoid almost all brands of crackers. If you want to prevent cancer you will strike these foods off your shopping list entirely.

Don't despair. There are some low fat brands of snacks and crackers that still taste good. Common examples are given in Table 7. Eat these in good health.

Table 6: Fat Content of High Fat Snacks

Avoid These

Brand	% Fat Calories
Potato Chips	
Pringles Regular	69%
Ruffles Regular	58%
Lays	58%
Health Valley	57%
Keebler Tato Skins	43%
Pringles Light	43%
Tortilla Chips	
Doritos Cool Ranch	49%
Hain Sesame	48%
Doritos	46%
Snyders	44%
Doritos Light	30%
Corn Chips	
Health Valley	62%
Planters	56%
Fritos	56%
Fritos Bar-B-Q	54%
Puffs	
Barbara's Cheese	68%
Cheetos Puffs	56%
Health Valley Cheese	55%
Cheetos Light	45%
Weight Watchers	45%

Table 7: Fat Content of Low Fat Snacks

Eat These

Brand	% Fat Calories
Breadsticks	
Wholewheat various brands	5% - 15%
Crackers	
Ak Mak Original	18%
Pretzels	
Snyders Old Fashioned	0%
Gibbles Old Fashioned	9%
Snyders Cheese	10%
Keebler Butter Nibblers	11%
Snyders Stix	11%
Bachman's Thin'n'Light	15%
Barbara's 9 grain	16%
Barbara's Whole Wheat	22%
Rice Cakes	
Quaker Rice Cakes	0%
Chico San Rice Cakes	0%
Mini Rice Cakes	0%
American Grains Rice Bites	25%

Source: Colgan Institute, Encinitas, CA

Chapter 8

High Fiber Prevents Cancer

America has very high rates of colon and rectal cancers. The National Cancer Institute predicts over 150,000 new cases for 1989. Many of these cancers are caused by faulty nutrition.

A comparison of diet and the incidence of colon and rectal cancers in twenty different countries, shows that all countries with high incidence eat a high-fat, low-fiber diet. All countries with low incidence eat a low-fat, high-fiber diet (28).

Uruguay and Argentina, for example, both eat a high beef, low fiber diet (like America). They have enormous rates of colorectal cancers. Neighboring South American countries that have small meat supplies, and eat far more grains, have very low rates (29).

Colon and rectal cancers develop from many interrelated causes, not just the fat level in the diet. Fiber is a big plus for prevention. The body expels many carcinogens in feces. The longer they remain in the bowel, the greater the risk of these carcinogens causing cancerous cell changes in the bowel lining. A high fiber diet can reduce the transit time of feces by up to 50% (30).

Fiber also acts to bind carcinogens in the intestines, making them less active, and giving them less access to the intestinal wall. It may also assist in normalizing the intestinal flora so that they produce fewer carcinogens (30a, 30b).

The same goes for bile acids. The liver excretes bile acids into the intestines for elimination. Recent studies show how bacteria act on these acids to produce carcinogens in combination with food wastes. These carcinogens then attack the walls of the bowel. The longer they remain, the higher the risk. By speeding transit time, and by absorbing bile acids, a high-fiber diet reduces this risk substantially. (31).

In the latest study, just published in the September, 1989 edition of the *Journal of the National Cancer Institute,* fiber has been shown to combat colorectal cancer directly. Dr. Jerome De Cosse at the New York Hospital, Cornell Medical Center, selected 58 people at high risk for colorectal cancer, who already had precancerous polyps growing in the rectal area. For four years, half the patients ate cereal twice daily, containing a daily total of 22.5 grams of fiber, mostly insoluble wheat bran. The other half of the patient sample ate a similar looking, but low-fiber cereal twice a day.

Compliance with the diet was monitered by a social worker. Results showed clearly that the precancerous polyps of the low fiber group continued to develop towards cancer. In sharp contrast, those who adhered to the high fiber diet, had fewer and smaller polyps than when they started four years earlier (31a).

These important new discoveries about fiber stem from pioneering work by Dr Dennis Burkitt in Britain in the 1960's. For many years they were not accepted by the US National Cancer Institute. Now, in a special addendum to a recent publication, NCI states:

> *Recent studies indicate that foods high in fiber — fruits and vegetables, peas and beans, whole grain breads and cereals — protect against some cancers, particularly colorectal (5).*

When people first come to the Colgan Institute, our records show that over the last 15 years and 30,000 subjects, they eat an average of only 19 grams of fiber a day. This low intake agrees with the National Cancer Institute figure for average American consumption of fiber, that is, 10-20 grams a day (5).

NCI recommends 25-35 grams of fiber daily (5). The Colgan Institute recommends 40-50 grams. In case you are unsure about fiber content of foods, Table 8 gives a list of foods and portions, each of which contains 10 grams of fiber. Four servings from this list daily will fill your fiber needs.

Table 8: Fiber "10"	
Each Item Contains 10 Grams of Dietary Fiber Aim for 40 - 50 Grams Per Day	
Grains	1/2 cup All Bran 1 cup Rolled Oats 1 cup Whole Grain Cereal 2 cobs Sweet Corn 3 Slices Whole Rye Bread 3 cups Puffed Wheat 4 oz. bag Popcorn
Vegetables	1/2 cup Mixed Beans 1/2 cup Peas, Lentils 1 cup Peanuts 2 cups Soybeans 2 cups steamed Vegetables 4 servings Mixed Salad 4 Carrots
Fruits	3 Pears 3 Bananas 4 Peaches 4 oz. Blueberries 5 Apples 6 Oranges 6 Dried Pear Halves 10 Dried Figs 20 Prunes 20 Dried Apricots

Source: Colgan Institute, Encinitas, CA

Chapter 9

Vegetables Prevent Cancer

A new development in cancer prevention, is the discovery that fruits and vegetables prevent cancer. Most people react to such a statement by, "Sure, vegetables are good for your health". But they don't know how good, or why. If it seems incredible to you that simple, everyday items, like cabbage, string beans, and carrots are more powerful against cancer than all the high-tech chemotherapy, let us examine a little of the evidence.

Recent studies have identified five major classes of compounds that occur in fruits and vegetables that are natural blocking agents against carcinogens. They are phenols, indoles, flavones, coumarins, and aromatic isothiocyanates (32). These blocking agents act by preventing carcinogens from reaching critical target sites for cancer.

There are also compounds in plants that prevent formation of carcinogens, such as ascorbic acid (vitamin C) and alpha tocopherol (vitamin E). These neutralizers of carcinogens are almost all vitamins or minerals or their co-factors. We will discuss them in subsequent chapters.

Finally, there are compounds in vegetables that act to reduce or eliminate cancers that have already formed. Again these are usually nutrients, such as vitamin A, and will be covered later. Here we are concerned only with blocking agents.

Various kinds of phenols occur in edible plants, including one that is now sold as a sports supplement. It is 4-hydroxy-3-methoxy cinnamic acid. The popular name is ferulic acid, which is the major active substance in gamma oryzanol, a compound extracted from rice bran oil. Ferulic acid and at least two other plant phenols have been shown to inhibit stomach cancer deliberately induced in mice (26).

The next category is indoles. Three indoles occur widely in cruciferous vegetables such as cabbage, cauliflower, broccoli, and brussels sprouts. These compounds inhibit stomach cancer and mammary cancer induced in animals (33,34).

Flavones, commonly called bioflavonoids also inhibit cancer. Common types are rutin, quercetin and tangeretin. They occur in numerous fruits. In animal studies they have shown powerful inhibitory effects on induced cancers (35).

Coumarins occur in a very wide variety of fruits and vegetables. Animal studies show that coumarins are potent inhibitors of induced mammary cancer, and moderate inhibitors of induced stomach cancer (36).

The final category of natural cancer blocking agents is aromatic isothiocyanates. Those tested against cancer occur mainly in cruciferous vegetables, including cabbage, cauliflower, broccoli and brussel sprouts. They have been shown to inhibit breast cancer, lung cancer and stomach cancer in animals. (37).

Much of this important work with vegetable inhibitors of cancer, has been completed in the last 10 years by Dr Lee Wattenberg and colleagues of the University of Minnesota Medical School. Consequently, it has not yet made its way through the ponderous bureaucracy of the National Cancer Institute to appear in their public recommendations, beyond vague advice to eat more produce.

In fact, NCI and other health agencies have been woefully unsuccessful in persuading Americans to eat fruit and vegetables. In over 20 years of "trying", our produce consumption rate has risen by only 7%.

The recommended intake of fruit and vegetables is four servings a day. Dr Gladys Block and colleagues at NCI have just completed a survey, showing that Americans actually eat, on average, **less than one serving a day of either fruit or vegetables** (potatoes and lettuce excluded) (38).

At the Colgan Institute, when people first come to us, their intake is similar to subjects in Dr Block's study. They eat less than one serving of fruit and vegetables daily (excluding canned food). One category of athletes is an exception. At first interview with us, bodybuilders score a daily average of 2.14 servings of vegetables and 1.5 servings of fruits.

This emphasis on produce is a definite protection against cancer. Now, in 1989, the American Cancer Society is trying to educate the public with what science has known for two decades. They have a new publication called **Cancer: Reduce Your Risk**, which advocates a high produce diet. The main vegetables and fruits containing good levels of substances proven to inhibit cancer are listed in Table 9.

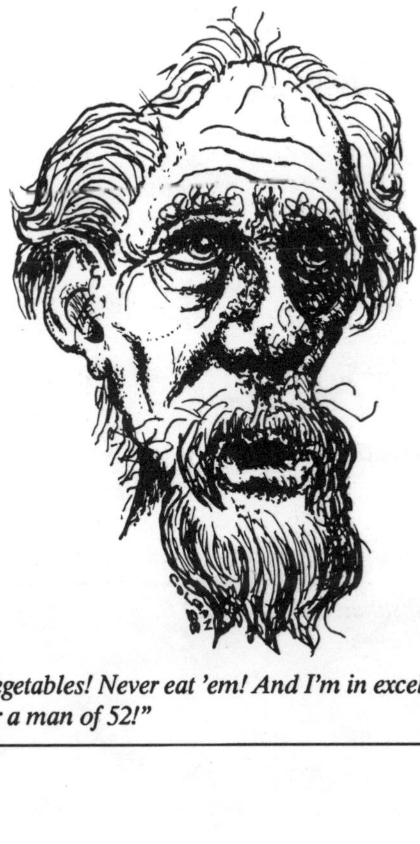

"Vegetables! Never eat 'em! And I'm in excellent health for a man of 52!"

Table 9: Anti-Carcinogenic Produce	
Vegetables	**Fruit**
Cabbages	Oranges
Cauliflower	Tangerines
Broccoli	Grapefruit
Brussels Sprouts	Papayas
Kale	Lemons
Squash	Uglis
Carrots	Persimmons
Green Beans	Mangos
Peppers	Peaches
Yams	Apricots

Source: Colgan Institute, Encinitas, CA

Chapter 10

Refined Foods Promote Cancer

White bread doesn't cause cancer directly. It's problem, and the problem of all refined flours, is that during processing they lose the nutrients required for their metabolism in the human body. Most white flour products, which covers the majority of breads and baked goods, are so devoid of nutrients that even weevils cannot live on them. And if weevils or other animals cannot be healthy on a food, neither can you.

What about "enriched" flour? Surely that is healthy with all those vitamins added to it. Wrong! Any college textbook of nutrition (38a) will tell you that human metabolism of carbohydrate requires the following vitamins and minerals:

thiamin
riboflavin
niacin
pantothenic acid
pyridoxine
phosphorus
magnesium

If even one of these nutrients is not present in adequate

amounts, the body cannot use the carbohydrate.

Virtually all of the eight nutrients are lost in the processing of white flour. Only three, thiamin, niacin, and riboflavin, are added back in so-called *enriched* flour. So, in order to use enriched flour breads and baked goods, the body has to rob itself, depriving nerves and muscles of pantothenic acid, depleting bones and heart of phosphorus and magnesium, and draining blood and brain of pyridoxine. In this way, high use of processed foods creates degenerative processes in the body that indirectly prepare it for cancer.

If this sounds like exageration, consider studies done by nutrition expert Professor Roger Williams and his colleagues at the University of Texas. They fed one group of young rats enriched bread. They fed a second group the same bread, plus a complete supply of vitamins and minerals. After three months, two-thirds of the enriched bread group had died, and the remainder had a variety of health problems. The rats given the additional vitamins and minerals all thrived (38b).

White bread is even worse. In another study, a group of rats fed on regular commercial white bread were all dead within 60 days (38c). If white flour foods cannot support as tough and adaptable a creature as a rat, you have no chance of being healthy on it. You are simply laying the base for degenerative disease. Cancer is the grimmest degenerative disease, always there waiting for an opportunity to proliferate.

What's the solution? In agreement with advice from the National Cancer Institute (5), the only sensible course is to strike white flour and enriched flour from your shopping list. Buy only whole grains, stone-ground, and certified organic. The best whole grains are listed in Table 10. Legumes are given also to mix with grains to complement their low levels of some amino acids, so as to make up complete proteins.

Caution. Many breads and baked goods called "whole wheat" or "whole grain" are not. When you read the ant size letters of the ingredients list, whole wheat maybe the third or fourth ingredient, or not there at all.

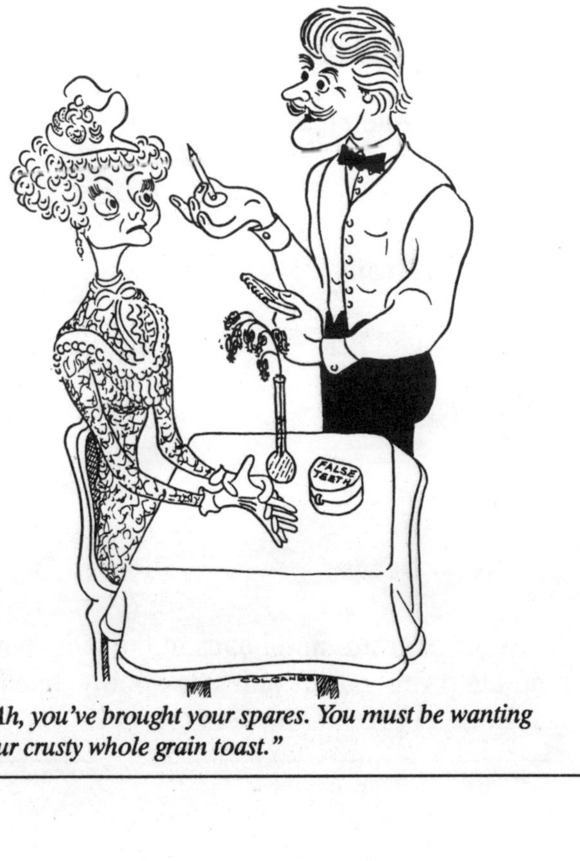

"Ah, you've brought your spares. You must be wanting our crusty whole grain toast."

Table 10: Top Twenty Grains and Legumes	
Best Protein Sources	**Best Carbohydrate Sources**
Over 20% Protein Under 20% Fat	**Under 5% Fat Over 70% Carbohydrate**
Soybeans	Brown Rice
Split Peas	Whole Barley
Kidney Beans	Whole Buckwheat
Dried Whole Peas	Whole Rye
Wheatgerm	Foxtail Millet
Lima Beans	Wild Rice
Black-eyed Peas	Whole Corn
Lentils	Pearl Millet
Black Beans	Whole Wheat
Navy Beans	Rolled Oats

A mixture of grains and beans in the diet provides complete proteins, but of lesser quality than fish, meat or dairy product proteins.

Source: Colgan Institute, Encinitas, CA

Chapter 11

Vitamins and Minerals Prevent Cancer

Taking vitamins and minerals as an anti-cancer strategy is still controversial. But even the highly conservative National Cancer Institute can no longer ignore the evidence. To quote from one of their publications: "*Studies indicate that vitamin A and vitamin C may help protect the body from some types of cancer.*" (5).

Of course, NCI suggests you can get these vitamins from foods, especially fruits and vegetables. So you can, and I hope you do. But most Americans don't eat nearly enough produce, as I showed in Chapter 9 by citing government studies. Other government studies show directly, that the general public is deficient in the very nutrients that NCI say may protect the body from cancer.

The government Health and Nutrition Examination Survey studied 28,000 people from age one through 74 in sixty-five different areas throughout the

United States. They examinined not only the diets people ate, but also the levels of nutrients in their blood (39). I will take some examples from this survey from the data on vitamins A and C, to show how the advice of NCI is just not working.

In the survey, one man in every four in Texas and in Washington State was deficient in vitamin A. One woman in every three was deficient in vitamin A. In various states, approximately 10% of all subjects were deficient in vitamin C, despite the addition of this vitamin to a wide range of foods and beverages. Overall, more that 60% of the people studied had at least one nutrient deficit.

Don't forget that these people were judged deficient even at the miniscule levels of intake that make up the US Recommended Dietary Allowances. These are levels formulated for the purpose of preventing specific nutrient deficiency diseases, such as scurvy from vitamin C deficiency. They are nowhere near the levels that may be necessary to prevent cancer.

A more recent study showed similar results. The Nationwide Food Consumption Survey of 15,000 households found that one in three ate diets deficient in calcium and vitamin B_6. One in every five households ate diets deficient in iron and vitamin A (39a).

A later report from the USDA analyzed 37,785 people. It examined intakes of only 11 of the essential nutrients. Results showed that the vast majority of subjects ate less than the RDA of Vitamins A and B_6 and minerals, calcium, iron and magnesium (39b). The percentages of people receiving insufficient nutrients are shown in Table 11. Because the sample was large and representative, similar percentages of nutrient deficiency are likely throughout the U.S. population.

Intake of other essential nutrients is equally dismal. The most recent government survey shows that 90% of Americans get inadequate amounts of the essential element chromium. The average daily intake is 33 micrograms for men and 25 micrograms for women (39c). The Food and Nutrition Board of U S National Academy of Sciences recommends 50 - 200 micrograms per day for normal health (39d).

The essential element zinc is also commonly deficient. In a study reported in the USRDA handbook, zinc in self-chosen diets of free living adults averaged only 8.6 milligrams/day (39e). The RDA for zinc is 15 mg/day, so it is likely that many people do not get sufficient for normal health (39d).

In the face of all this evidence, some conservative factions of the medical profession still insist that we get all the vitamins and minerals we need from our food. In my lectures to these physicians, I find that most of them don't know the research, and are also uninformed about the poor state of American food. Once they read the studies, many change their minds. If you are not convinced, then read the references cited, plus two other publications of mine, *Your Personal Vitamin Profile* (Morrow) (40), and *Effects of Multi-nutrient Supplementation on Athletic Performance* (Human Kinetics) (41). Then, no matter who tries to tell you vitamins are unnecessary, you will know better.

Table 11: Nutrient Intake of Sample of 37,785 U. S. Citizens

Nutrient	% receiving less than the full RDA	% receiving the full RDA or more
Vitamin B6	80	20
Magnesium	75	25
Calcium	68	32
Iron	57	43
Vitamin A	50	50
Thiamin	45	55
Vitamin C	41	59
Riboflavin	34	66
Vitamin B12	34	66
Niacin	33	67
Phosphorus	27	73

Source: United States Department of Agriculture, (39b)

Food Degradation

How did our diet go so wrong, from the wonderful whole grains, organic produce and lean, free range meat of our forefathers? Studies show clearly that the food supply has been progressively degraded since 1860 by heavier and heavier loading of foods with nutritionally empty fats and sugars. In the 1860's we ate 53% complex carbohydrates, 10% simple sugars and only 25% fats. By 1975 complex carbohydrates had fallen to only 22%, sugars more than doubled to 24%, and fats jumped to 42% (41a). Much of this excess sugar and fat is highly processed and devoid of nutrients.

The second major cause of loss of nutrients in our diet is soil depletion. With the advent of chemical fertilization, most farm soils in America became overused and stripped of numerous essential minerals. In farming the focus is on producing healthy crops, not on producing healthy people.

Depleted soils will grow fine-looking crops if fertilized with only phosphorus, potassium and nitrogen. But bodies are not vegetables.Human health requires, in addition, calcium, chromium, zinc, selenium, iodine, manganese, magnesium, molybdenum, iron, copper, cobalt, boron, fluoride, nickel and vanadium. These have been progressively depleted in American farm soils since the 1920's.

The third source of loss of nutrients in foods is modern processing, the hazardous journey of food today from field to table. To take a few examples from the American Medical Association's Council on Food and Nutrition, lettuce loses half it's vitamin C if kept a mere three days in the refrigerator. Asparagus, broccoli and green beans lose half their vitamin C in cold storage before they reach your greengrocer. Cooking these vegetables destroys another 25% of their vitamin C, plus up to 70% of their thiamin, and 50% of their riboflavin (41b). And we call this "fresh" produce.

If you can the produce, results are worse. Renowned authority on nutrients in food, Dr. Henry Schroeder has shown that canning carrots removes 70% of their cobalt; canning tomatoes removes 80% of their zinc. Canning of green vegetables destroys more than half their contents of B vitamins. Dr. Schroeder reports similar losses for hundreds of foods (41c).

Let us put these five lines of evidence together. First, government studies show widespread nutrient deficiencies in American diets. Second, government studies show widespread nutrient deficiencies in American bodies. Third, the composition of the diet has progressively deteriorated since 1860, so that now it is loaded with nutritionally empty fats and sugars. Fourth, synthetic fertilization has depleted farm soils of essential minerals. Fifth, modern processing destroys much of the nutrient content of foods.

Together, these facts are a strong indication that you cannot rely on your food to provide the nutrients to protect you from cancer. Nutrient supplementation seems the only sensible way.

Good Vitamins, Bad Vitamins

The next problem is finding appropriate multivitamins and minerals. Yes, there are hundreds of brands but very, very few good ones. In America, vitamins come under the food regulations. They are not pharmaceuticals. Anyone can go to a manufacturer and have any formula they like made up. No permit is required, no FDA approval, no tests, no licenses, no bona fides at all.

The Colgan Institute has designed hundreds of formulations for a huge range of companies. Often the main request is to design a pill to a certain price, to fit a certain market niche. We refuse these requests and design only to fit human health. But, by the time the pill hits the market, almost inevitably our formulation has been watered down and changed to reduce costs. Often it has become next to useless as a nutritional aid.

Good but expensive forms of minerals, such as ascorbates and picolinates, are replaced by cheap oxides and sulfates that most human bodies can barely use at all. Very expensive nutrients like biotin are cut to a few micrograms (millionths of a gram), reducing their biological effectiveness almost to zero. Other essential nutrients, such as linolenic acid are left out altogether, because they are difficult to deal with chemically, and reduce the shelf life of the product.

And I am talking about the good guys, companies prepared to pay high fees to consultants like the **Colgan Institute** to design the best for them. We never see the bad guys, who litter the market with miracle pills, different ones every year, designed on a scratch pad in the executive lunchroom to take advantage of the latest market buzz words.

To help you avoid these scams, Table 12 lists the daily levels of nutrients used by the Colgan Institute as **a base formula**. It cannot provide for the wide individual differences in nutrient needs, but at least it offers a base from which you can judge other products. Two companies that make top quality multi-nutrient supplements are Nutrition Research Laboratories of San Diego (619) 632-7722, and TwinLabs of Ronkonkoma, New York (516) 467-3140.

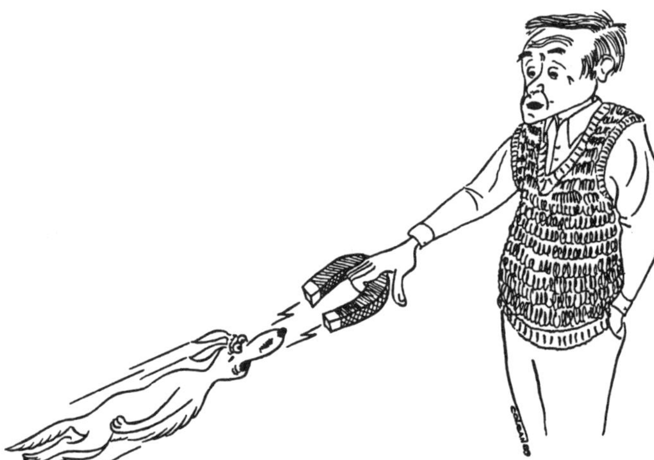

"Honey, I've found your iron pills."

Table 12: Multi-Vitamin/Mineral Basic Formula

Fat Soluble Vitamins	
Vitamin A	
Beta-carotene	12,500 I.U.
Retinol	7,500 I.U
Vitamin D3 (Cholecalciferol)	400 I.U.
Vitamin E (D, alpha-tocopherol)	300 I.U.
Vitamin K (Phylloquinone)	75 mcg.
Water Soluble Vitamins	
Vitamin B_1 (Thiamin)	25 mg
Vitamin B_2 (Riboflavin)	25 mg
Vitamin B_3 (Niacin)	30 mg
(Niacinamide)	40 mg
Vitamin B_5 (Pantothenic acid)	50 mg
Vitamin B_6 (Pyridoxine)	25 mg
Vitamin B12 (Cobalamin)	50 mg
Biotin	500 mcg
Folic Acid	400 mcg
Vitamin C (Ascorbic acid)	50 mg
(Calcium ascorbate)	150 mg
(Ascorbyl palmitate)	50 mg
(Magnesium ascorbate)	50 mg
Essential Fatty Acids	
Linoleic Acid	150 mg
Linolenic Acid	150 mg
Gamma Linolenic Acid	25 mg

Continued on page 62

Table 12: Continued

Lipogenics	
Choline	50 mg
Inositol	50 mg
Accessory Nutrients	
Coenzyme Q10	30 mg
Para-amino-benzoic acid	35 mg
Citrus Bioflavonoids	150 mg
Minerals*	
Calcium (carbonate)	800 mg
Magnesium (aspartate)	600 mg
Potassium (aspartate)	100 mg
Iron (picolinate)	10 mg
Zinc (picolinate)	15 mg
Manganese (gluconate)	5 mg
Boron (aspartate)	3 mg
Copper (gluconate)	500 mcg
Chromium (picolinate)	200 mcg
Selenium (Selenomethionine)	200 mcg
Iodine (Potassium iodide)	100 mcg
Molybdenum (trioxide)	40 mcg

*Mineral amounts given are elemental, that is actual amounts of the element itself, not the amounts of the compound in which the element is provided. For example, calcium carbonate is only 40% calcium. So to provide 800 mg of calcium, you require 2,000 mg of calcium carbonate.

Source: Colgan Institute, Encinitas, CA

Chapter 12

Antioxidents Prevent Cancer

The newest development in cancer prevention is the use of high levels of antioxidant nutrients. To date, the National Cancer Institute and other health authorities, have not directly recommended antioxidants as a class of cancer preventatives. They have recommended individual antioxidant nutrients, namely vitamin A, beta carotene, vitamin C and vitamin E. To these, other cancer researchers add selenium, L-glutathione and co-enzyme Q10.

The evidence that these antioxidants prevent cancer is now irrefutable. In the last decade, hundreds of studies have confirmed it, including studies by the National Cancer Institute.

Currently NCI is funding over thirty different studies on cancer inhibiting effects of a wide variety of antioxidant nutrients. But it may take until the turn of the century before they make any definite recommendations. I want to give you some of the latest findings now, so you can check the references and decide for yourself, a decade in advance of bureaucracy.

Vitamin C Prevents Cancer

For vitamin C, cancer expert Dr Bruce Ames of the University of California, Berkeley, reviews a mass of animal studies showing strong inhibitory effects by vitamin C on a variety of cancers. (42). Human evidence is more sparse, but the work of Dr Linus Pauling and Dr Ewan Cameron shows decisively, that large intakes of vitamin C can inhibit the growth of existing cancers in human patients (43).

Linus Pauling is too controversial for some "*establishment*" people, who ousted the double Nobel laureate from their ranks when he first proposed using large supplements of vitamin C in the 1960's. Since then the Colgan Institute has reviewed hundreds of studies worldwide that absolutely support Pauling. We are pleased to give him due credit for alerting us all to the power of vitamin C.

Dr E Bjelke, for example, did extensive studies at the University of Minnesota, of almost 5,000 men in America and 8,000 men in Norway. He found that those with a high intake of vitamin C, had much lower incidence of cancer of the stomach, colon and rectum (44).

A lot of these cancers are caused by regular food. Substances in your food, especially nitrates and nitrites, cause the body to form potent carcinogens in the gut, called nitrosamines. Even though we know this, nitrites are still added as preservatives to numerous foods. On a single visit to a local supermarket, staff of the Colgan Institute compiled a list of 71 foods with added nitrites. With this level of food pollution, its a good bet you have nitrites in your diet too.

One way that vitamin C prevents cancer is by stopping nitrosamines from forming in the gut. Dr D Wagner and colleagues, for example, have shown that two grams of vitamin C can block nitrosamine formation from ingested nitrites by 81% (45).

That is not all that vitamin C does. Important recent work by Drs William Benedict and Peter Jones at the University of Southern California, School of Medicine, has shown that ascorbic acid can completely protect cells that have been exposed to the potent carcinogen 3-methylcholanthrene. Better still, ascorbate can **reverse** cancerous changes that have previously been induced in cell cultures (45a).

Extrapolating from numerous in vitro and animal studies to the human case, the daily amounts of vitamin C required are in the gram range. It is not possible to obtain these amounts from regular food. Supplementation is the only way.

"But", say the critics,"that is so unnatural, taking pills your whole life." Sadly, gentlemen, man has created an unnatural, toxic environment in which he now has to live. Taking concentrated nutrients in pill form is indeed unnatural, but no more so than breathing the carcinogenic fumes of industrial wastes that smog the dawn of every city day.

Vitamin E Prevents Cancer

Strong evidence also supports vitamin E as a cancer preventative.. In 1988, Dr P Knekt and colleagues in Finland reported the latest long-term study. They followed 21,000 men for 10 years. Men with high vitamin E intake, and high blood levels of vitamin E, had a 30% lower risk for all types of cancer (46).

In a second study, Dr. Knekt followed 15,000 women for eight years, all initially free of cancer. During the follow-up, women with low serum vitamin E developed cancer 1.6 times more frequently than women with high serum vitamin E (46a).

The mineral selenium is synergistic with vitamin E in it's anti-cancer effects. In the Knekt study, women with low serum vitamin E **and** low serum selenium had **10 times** the risk of breast cancer. In animal studies where breast cancer is deliberately induced, combined supplementation with vitamin E and selenium protects more animals than either nutrient used alone (46b).

Lung cancer, the leading cancer risk, is also related to vitamin E. One recent study by Dr. M Menkes and colleagues followed large groups of subjects, 88 of whom subsequently developed lung cancer. These patients showed significantly lower blood levels of vitamin E than controls (46c).

Like vitamin C, the amount of vitamin E that may be required to prevent cancer is larger than can be provided by regular food. One recent recommendation in the conservative *Journal of the American Dietetic Association* is 200-800 I. U. per day (46d).

Vitamin A Prevents Cancer

In an authoritative review of all major studies, Drs Thomas Kummet and Frank Meyskins of the University of Arizona concluded, "*a protective effect of vitamin A has has been found for almost all sites of cancer*" (47).

Most human studies of vitamin A have measured intake of beta-carotene, as much as they have vitamin A, because diets in Western Society derive more than half their vitamin A from carotenoids. Multiple studies now show that beta-carotene has a stronger protective effect than straight vitamin A (48,49). A fortunate finding, because high intakes of vitamin A can be very toxic, whereas beta-carotenc has low toxicity.

The biggest dietary study of beta carotene was done in Japan on 250,000 people, as part of the 1965 census. After 10 years 7,377 had developed cancer. The analysis showed, that those whose diets were low in beta carotene, had increased risk of cancer of the lung, stomach, colon, prostate and cervix (48a).

Some scientists remain unconvinced by these epidemiological studies. There always seems to be the possibility of bias in analyzing people's diets. Fortunately, there is now direct evidence that vitamin A and beta carotene prevent cancer. One important study, reported in the leading British medical journal, the *Lancet*, was done on betel nut chewers and tobacco chewers. Both habits are strongly linked with oral cancer. First the researchers measured the numbers of abnormal cells in the mouths of the chewers. Although these cells are not cancers, they are predictive of a pre-cancerous state. Then one group was given a daily supplement of vitamin A or beta carotene for twelve weeks. In unsupplemented chewers, the number of abnormal cells remained the same or increased slightly. In the supplemented chewers, abnormal cells were reduced by two-thirds (48b). There is no longer any doubt that vitamin A and beta carotene can prevent cancer.

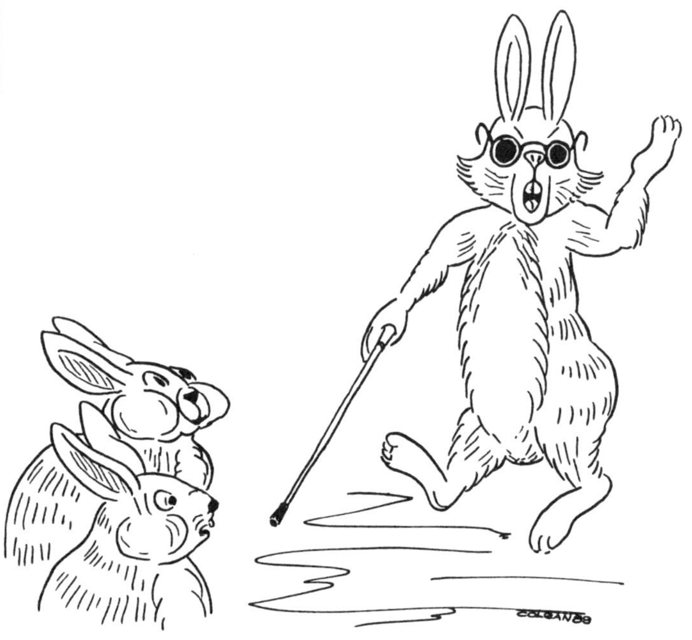

"Bugsy gave up carrots when he heard beta carotene might be toxic."

Selenium Prevents Cancer

Cancer expert, Professor Bruce Ames, head of the Department of Biochemistry at Berkely, reviews numerous animal studies showing that dietary supplements of selenium inhibit developments of deliberately induced cancers of the breast, liver, skin and colon (48c).

Epidemiological studies of human subjects reinforce this evidence. Between 1968 and 1972, Dr Paul Knekt and colleagues in Finland took and froze serum samples from 21,172 men. Over the next decade, 143 developed lung cancer. The stored serums were then analyzed and compared with the serums of a control group. The cancer victims showed much lower serum selenium levels than the controls. Subjects with low selenium levels had three times the risk of subsequent lung cancer (48d). The study concluded that inadequate selenium nutrition is a high risk factor for lung cancer.

Selenium deficiency does not only affect the lungs. Dr. V Reinhold and colleagues in the Department of Dermatology at the University of Bonn have found similar effects in the deadly skin cancer melanoma. They examined the serum of 101 melanoma patients and compared it with controls. The patients showed significantly lower levels of selenium, even in early stages of the disease.

These findings indicate that the deficient selenium nutrition **preceded** the melanoma. Selenium is known to protect skin from ultra-violet damage. So it is likely that the deficit was a primary cause of the cancer (48e).

This study is especially important because of the loss of part of the ozone layer protecting the Earth from untra-violet light, caused by our worldwide careless use of chlorofluorocarbons. The Environmental Protection Agency predicts over one million additional cases of skin cancer in America before the end of the century caused directly by the depletion of ozone. No one can protect you except yourself. It seems only common sense to ensure that you have an adequate intake of selenium.

How much is adequate? A difficult question because selenium can be very toxic even at a daily intake of one milligram. The National Academy of Sciences suggests 50-200 micrograms as safe and sensible for normal nutrition (48f).

They suggest that that amount can be obtained from a good varied diet. I do not agree. In 1981 I published a short report in *Science* indicating that selenium is deficient in the soils of most of Connecticut, Delaware, Illinois, Indiana, Massachusetts, New York, Ohio, Oregon, Pennsylvania, Rhode Island and the District of Columbia. If the soil is deficient, then so is the meat and the produce you eat, and therefore, so are you. The Colgan Institute routinely uses 200-400 micrograms of supplemental selenium in the organically bound selenomethionine form.

Glutathione Prevents Cancer

Your body makes glutathione continuously from the amino acids cysteine and methonine. L-glutathione is one of your main endogenous (in the body) antioxidants. It is probably the main cellular defense against alkylating and oxidative carcinogens (48g). This discovery may be vital to our understanding of cancer and other degenerative diseases, because glutathione levels decline with aging equally in mosquito, mouse and man (48j).

What happens when you stop this decline? At the Department of Biochemistry of the University of Louisville School of Medicine, Professor Calvin Lang and colleagues gave mosquitoes supplemental precursors of glutathione. Their glutathione levels shot up, and their lifespan was extended by a whopping **40%** (48h).

Now, a mosquito is not a good model for a man, but what about a mouse. Drs Jaime Miguel and Hans Weber of the Alexander Medical Foundation in San Carlos, CA gave mice the same precursor of glutathione, a compound called thiazolidine-4-carboxylic acid (TC for short). In TC treated animals, glutathione went up and lifespan was extended (48k).

In the human case, no one has yet studied the lifetime effects of glutathione supplementation. We do know, however, that chronologically old people who maintain high blood levels of glutathione, suffer fewer diseases and score as biologically much younger than their age (48j).

The evidence points strongly to glutathione as an inhibitor of degenerative disease in general, as well as an anti-cancer agent in particular. There is even evidence that it can protect animals against aflatoxin, one of the most potent know carcinogens (481). No one knows the amount required to protect a man. Following an extensive review of all the studies, the Colgan Institute uses up to 250 mg per day of pre-formed L-glutathione. As far as we can determine, that should be enough.

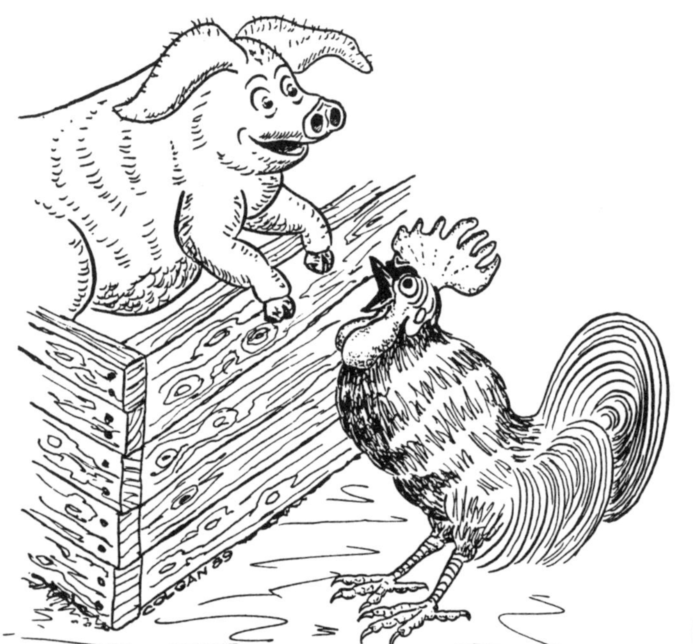

"Us fat hams are off the menu.
It's your skinny wives for the chop these days."

Coenzyme Q10 Prevents Cancer

Coenzyme Q10 is the most recent and probably the most controversial essential nutrient to be added to the list of potent antioxidants. Your body can't make coenzyme Q10. It is derived from Coenzyme Q, which occurs widely in foods, hence it's common name ubiquinone (from ubiquitous).

Despite this abundance, the level of coenzyme Q10 declines in the body with age. This decline has recently been traced to decline of an enzyme in the liver that converts Co Q to Co Q10 (48m).

There is very compelling evidence from animal studies that you should maintain a high level of Co Q10. In one study, Dr Emile Bliznakov and colleagues at the New England Research Institute in Connecticut induced cancer in mice by injection of dibenzpyrene, the most potent carcinogen in tobacco. One group of mice was given a diet supplemented with Co Q10. The rest were given just the diet. Ten weeks later every one of the unsupplemented mice had developed tumors. One quarter of the supplemented mice never developed tumors for the duration of the study (48m).

Co Q10 has been a widely used nutrient in Japanese medicine since 1980. It is only now coming into use in America. Amounts required to inhibit cancer are unknown. Since 1985 The Colgan Institute has used supplements of 30-60 mg per day.

Chapter 13

Immunity Against Cancer

Antioxidants also prevent cancer by a second mechanism, even more powerful than their direct action to neutralize or prevent the formation of carcinogens. They also strengthen your most important defense against cancer -- your immune system.

This discovery has not yet percolated from the laboratories to the media, and may not become public knowledge until the turn of the century. But in the inner circles of nutrition science, the immunological benefits of antioxidants are now so well accepted, that many eminent scientists have adopted a daily routine of antioxidant supplementation. Why? Because boosting the immune system not only protects you from cancer, it protects you from everything.

Here are the bare bones facts. The breakthrough experiments were done in the early 1970s. Dr. Robert Tengerdy and colleagues at Colorado State University, discovered that supplementing animal diets with large amounts of vitamin E, protected them against various diseases and toxins deliberately introduced into their bodies. The basis of this protection was a big increase in immune strength (49a, 49b). The most important point of this discovery is that control animals, whose diets contained the equivalent of adequate amounts of vitamin E for humans, according to the USRDA, were not protected, and succumbed to disease.

Spallholtz and colleagues obtained the same effect by using the antioxidant co-factor, selenium (49c). In both sets of experiments, immune strength increased to four times the usual response -- **four times!** By 1981 Tengerdy and colleagues concluded that maintaining strong immunity may require **six times** the vitamin E previously thought to be adequate (49d).

These studies have since been confirmed in other laboratories (49e). They are most important in preventing cancer because they provide a new way to strengthen immunity. Many nutrients are involved in maintaining immunity, but they exert their action by effects on protein and nucleic acid metabolism (49f). Supplemental antioxidants, beyond the amounts needed for "normal" health, boost immunity by an entirely different mechanism.

To explain this mechanism we have to dip into a smidgen of basic science. Bear with me. It's worth it. Immunity is controlled by a vast army of specialized cells. I will take as an example one of the main divisions -- cell mediated immunity. In cell mediated immunity, our most important immune cells, the lymphocytes, you might say the cavalry, attack and destroy cancer cells by recognizing their foreign surface markings.

Then other immune cells, the infantry, called macrophages, move in and engulf the dead and dying cancer cells. In the process of their work, the macrophages themselves cause a lot of damage, mostly by making toxic oxidation products (49g). They weaken their own cavalry, the lymphocytes, thereby reducing their capacity to deal with new cancer cells. So, in acting against disease, the immune system also attacks itself (49h).

No one has yet worked out a comprehensive theory to explain this weakness in immune function. One of my forthcoming books, *Stop Aging* (Morrow), explains it in more detail, and contends it may be a fault in human evolution. Whatever the reality, it seems certain that large amounts of supplemental antioxidants are needed lifelong, to protect lymphocyte function against the toxins produced by the action of macrophages. We need to protect our immune army from it's own troops.

These discoveries are most important for prevention of cancer, because of the strong correlation between the decline of immunity with usual human aging, and the concomitant rapid rise of cancer risk. The ultimate key to cancer prevention is maintaining **host resistance.**

Does it work? Animal studies say yes. For example, in one type of laboratory mouse, the C3H mouse, 80% develop mammary cancer as they age, because of an endemic mammary tumor virus in the strain. By long term supplementation with selenium, incidence of mammary cancer is reduced to 10% (49j).

Because it is acting against a virus, the effect of the selenium is not as a simple antioxidant. The only way it can work is as a complex booster of immune function. The mechanisms of this beneficial effect remain to be discovered.

Selenium supplementation also increases the ability of experimental subjects to reject transplanted malignant tumors and tissue grafts from other animals. Both these effects are a result of strengthened immunity (49k).

Supporting the idea that antioxidants boost immunity directly, other studies show that antioxidant supplements given over long periods, prevent the decline of immunity with aging (49l). Finally, even when immunity has declined with age, supplementary antioxidants can restore it (49m).

I have presented only a small fraction of the evidence that antioxidants can prevent cancer, both by their actions to neutralize carcinogens and by their actions to boost immune function. The amounts required to do so in humans are yet unknown. So it is not possible to recommend daily amounts. The best estimate we can make to date is to extrapolate from animal studies to the human case, while maintaining a safety margin against any possible toxicity. Table 13 shows the extrapolated amounts of antioxidants that may be required to prevent cancer in a healthy person of average weight and normal metabolism.

Table 13. Daily amounts of Antioxidants Used to Prevent Animal Cancers (extrapolated to the human case)

Antioxidant Nutrient	Daily Intake
Vitamin C	2000 - 12,000 mg
Vitamin E	400 - 1,600 I.U.
Selenium* (organically bound)	200 - 400 mcg
L-glutathione	50 - 250 mg
Zinc**	20 - 70 mg
Coenzyme Q10	30 - 60 mg
Beta-carotene***	5,000 - 25,000 I.U.

*Selenium can become very toxic at over 800 micrograms per day, especially in the inorganic form of sodium selenite.

** Zinc acts as an antioxidant co-factor.

***Beta-carotene is a safe source of vitamin A at the levels given. Vitamin A may become toxic beyond 25,000 I.U. per day

Source: Colgan Institute, Encinitas, CA

Chapter 14

Essential Fatty Acids Prevent Cancer

Popular media have not latched onto essential fatty acids -- yet. So the public is not generally aware that there are two fats the body cannot make, but must have for good health -- linoleic acid and linolenic acid.

You have to get these fatty acids from your food. Today that's not so easy. Only a few common foods contain adequate amounts of both essential fatty acids. These are flax seeds, pumpkin and squash seeds, soybeans and walnuts. Cooking oils made from these seeds are also adequate, but only if they are truly cold pressed and otherwise unprocessed. That's the way our food used to be.

Not anymore. All mass produced oils in America today, including all margarines and cooking oils, are now processed to the extent that most of their essential fatty acids are destroyed (50).

In the fresh, cold pressed oil, the essential fatty acids are in a chemical form called a **cis** configuration.

This is the only form that can be used by the body. If you heat or hydrogenate these oils, or subject them to other chemical treatments, then the **cis** configuration is changed to a **trans** configuration. Trans fatty acids cannot function in the body as essential fats (50,51). They provide only excess empty calories, worse than useless in our corpulent land.

Only a few small companies still make real, cold pressed oils. Your best bet is fresh pumpkin seeds, soybeans or walnuts. A second alternative is extra virgin olive oil, the only readily available oil that is truly cold pressed. Extra virgin olive oil contains large amounts of cis linoleic acid, but no linolenic acid. To get your linolenic acid, or it's equivalent, you have to add cold water fish such as salmon, trout, mackerel and sardines.

These fish contain large amounts of the fish oils, docosahexanoic acid and eicosapentanoic acid. Both have the chemical make up termed omega-3. The body can use these in place of linolenic acid, which is also omega-3. Using extra virgin olive oil in your salads and general foods, and eating two meals of cold-water fish per week, should provide all the essential fatty acids you need.

What has this to do with cancer? The connection is new and still controversial because, as with vitamin and mineral deficiencies, the human body will keep going for a long time on inadequate supplies of fatty acids. But all the while you are deficient, degenerative processes are taking place in your body. Any degenerative process makes it easier for cancer to occur.

There is also some evidence that essential fatty acids can directly inhibit cancer. Dr Nola Dippenaar and colleagues at the Medical University of Southern Africa in Pretoria added gamma linolenic acid to cultures infected with cancer cells. The cancer cells died, and the cultures returned to normal (51b).

In intact animals, Dr R Tanure and colleagues fed one group of rats supplemental corn oil that contains zero omega-3 fatty acids. They fed a second group supplemental fish oil rich in omega-3. Afer a week they injected both groups with the carcinogen, 1, 2, -dimethylhydrazine, potent in causing colorectal cancer. The fish oil supplemented rats developed significantly fewer colorectal and gastrointestinal tumors (51c). In the latest study, Dr Colin Campbell of Cornell University showed that fish oil given to rats **after** precancerous cells had developed, significantly inhibited development of cancer(51d).

How specific fatty acids work to inhibit cancer is unknown. Likely it involves a delicate balance of substances called prostaglandins that regulate the internal chemistry of your cells. All we can say for sure is that the sort of disorganized cell growth that occurs in cancer, flourishes in a cellular environment where essential fatty acids are deficient, and the fats that are present lack the necessary biological activity to maintain normal cellular functions (51).

If you eat the usual cooking oils and margarines sold in supermarkets today, you are creating exactly the type of deficient fatty environment found in and around cancers. Strike them off your shopping list. Aim for the best of the cold pressed oils. Some health food stores sell unprocessed pumpkin seed, walnut or soybean oils. All contain both essential fatty acids. Otherwise use extra virgin olive oil and eat cold water fish. To help you in finding the best oils, Table 14 lists the good, the bad, and the downright ugly.

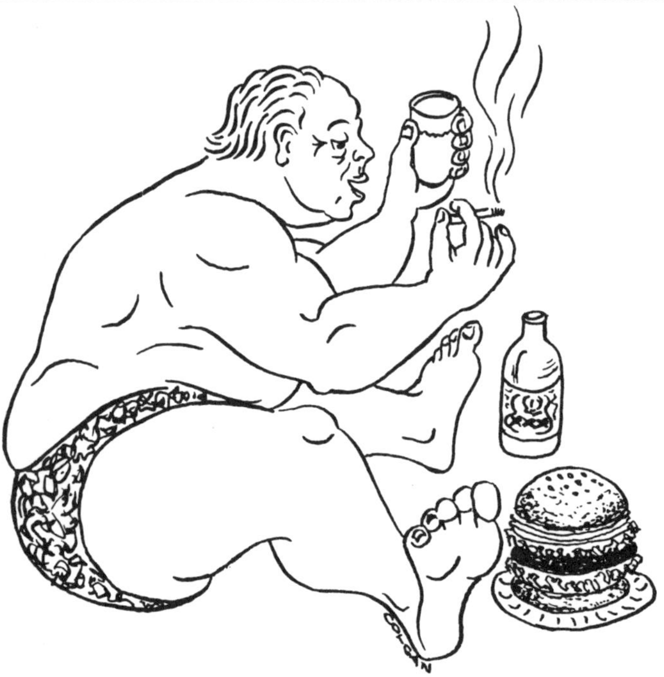

"You need plenty of fat in the burgers to save your throat from the cigarettes."

Table 14: Essential Fatty Acids in Oils*

Source	Linoleic Acid	Linolenic Acid	Saturated Fats
		Good Oils	
Cold Water Fish		High Omega 3	Low
Flax (Linseed)	15%	56%	9%
Pumpkin Seed	45%	15%	8%
Soybean	50%	10%	15%
Walnut	51%	5%	16%
		2nd Best	
Safflower	75%		12%
Sunflower	65%		12%
Sesame	45%		13%
Almond	17%		15%
Virgin Olive	8%		16%
Corn	59%		17%
		Bad Oils (both contain toxins)	
Peanut	30%		21%
Cottonseed	50%		26%
		Downright Ugly Oils	
Palm	11%		50%
Palm Kernal	2%		85%
Coconut	3%		91%

*Percentages for non hydrogenated cold pressed oils.

Canola (rapeseed) oil contains both essential fatty acids but is not included because of questions about it's content of toxic erucic acid.

Sources: Colgan Institute and Erasmus V, Fats and Oils (50).

Chapter 15

Don't Drink the Water

You are two-thirds water. It is the most important nutrient in your body. The average person consumes three-quarters of a gallon of water every day in foods and drinks. The quality of the water you consume affects every chemical reaction inside you.

Despite these clear facts, most Americans still drink faucet water and use it for cooking food. Almost all faucet water comes from polluted sources in rivers, streams and lakes (52.) In 1988, The U.S. Department of Public Health announced that 85% of American water is contaminated to a dangerous level. The Environmental Protection Agency states that 23 million Americans are drinking polluted water.

But don't they clean our water at the treatment stations? They try. To purify it, however, would be far too expensive, because 95% of the domestic water supply is not drunk at all. It goes down the drain in bathroom, sink and laundry. So it is cleaned only to the minimum standard required to prevent water borne disease (53).

Staff of the Colgan Institute carry water testers on lecture tours. We routinely measure the pollutants in drinking water in hotels, health clubs, restaurants and health conventions. To date we have found only one case where the water was pure (less that 20 ppm pollutants). Commonly we find levels of 300 - 700 ppm pollutants.

If you pollute every cell of your body from the water you drink, you can expect degeneration. The connection between polluted water and cancer is almost impossible to prove, but the connection between degeneration and cancer is clear. Cancer is the end product of long-term bodily degeneration. Don't allow it to happen to you.

Clean Your Water

You can buy bottled distilled water. But it becomes a heavy item in more ways than one in the weekly shopping basket. Delivered water is also expensive, and equally inconvenient, with all those bottles to tote. The best solution is an efficient water cleaning system at home.

In the near future, proper water cleaning systems will be a standard feature in new houses. They will have to be, because our water supply is getting dirtier every year. Currently, however, there are all sorts of what you might call transition products. These vary from simple carbon filters to very sophisticated copies of laboratory water cleaning systems. Prices go from \$50 to \$5,000. Water cleaning is a great case of caveat emptor (buyer beware). Most of the cheap filter systems remove only large particles and make the water taste a little better. They leave behind all the carcinogenic heavy metals, pesticide residues and other chemicals for you to drink. Some filters even contaminate the water further.

For example, between 1982 and 1986 Norelco sold many thousands of their "Clean Water Machine". The filter in this system was contaminated with methylene chloride, which polluted the very water it was supposed to clean. In 1987 the Colgan Institute tested five popular brands of water filters sold through health food stores, sports outlets and by multilevel marketing. Four of them left in most of the pollutants. Only one got the water clean enough to drink, the Seagull IV.

Much better are the new four-step reverse osmosis systems using Kodak's cellulose triacetate (CTA) membranes. They can remove up to 97% of contaminants. The Colgan Institute has tested one of these systems for more than a year. For water that starts at 500 ppm contaminants (a common level for city water), the system produces water at 20-40 ppm contaminants.

But reverse osmosis is not the best method. Far and away the cleanest water is produced by the new home distillers. Unlike the older models that required frequent cleaning and manual attention and lasted only 2-3 years, the latest distillers are no more trouble than your house furnace, and give constant clean water to faucets placed wherever you need them. They are built to last at least a decade.

One of the best is the Pure Water A-12 system

produced by Pure Water Inc. of Lincoln, Nebraska- (402) 467-9300. At the Colgan Institute, we have been running and testing one of them continuously for the last two years, producing 12 gallons of clean water per day. With entry water of 500+ ppm contaminants, it yields water of 2-12 ppm. That's about as clean as you can get.

As we go to press there is an advance on the A-12 called the D-3 from AR Systems, Hopewell, Va (804) 541-8802. It is a superb energy conserving design with automatic water cooling and multiple fail-safe systems for at least a decade of trouble free operation.

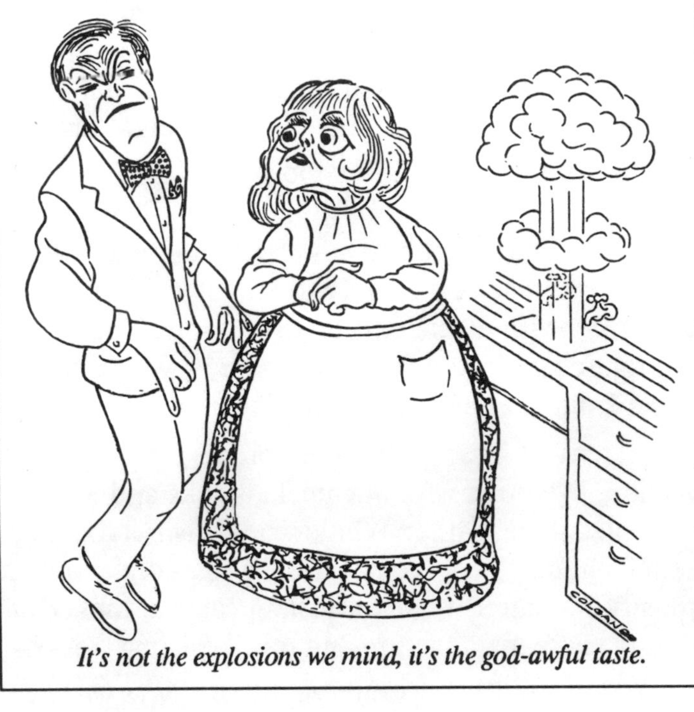

It's not the explosions we mind, it's the god-awful taste.

Chapter 16

Food Pollution Causes Cancer

Early in 1989, farm workers union leader Cesar Chavez went on a hunger strike, to protest the exposure of his members to the carcinogenic chemicals on grapes. Right after that we had the Alar on apples, an unnecessary pollutant used on red apples mainly to make them look prettier. The Environmental Protection Agency knew about the dangers of Alar since 1984, but didn't plan to ban it until 1992.

The general public was alerted to the problem in 1989, when actress Meryl Streep got wide publicity for her concern at the danger to children. The EPA's own figures indicated that 6,000 Americans could get cancer from Alar before it was withdrawn.

Tens of thousands of us protested the EPA's inaction, by voting with our pocketbooks and leaving red apples at the market. Whole school districts banned them from lunch counters. Running scared, the apple industry pressured Uniroyal Chemical, the maker of Alar, to cease manufacture and recall existing stocks.

One small victory but not the war. Now we have

heptachlor, a pesticide banned since 1978, turning up in 1989 in 400,000 Arkansas chickens. And, we have just learned from the EPA, that parathion, a known carcinogen, is widely used on broccoli, and residues cannot be washed off. A new report by Wildlife Federation scientist Dr Jeffery Foran in the *American Journal of Public Health* shows that all fish from the Great Lakes, including those delicious soho and chinook salmon, are polluted with levels of DDT and Deildrin that are dangerously carcinogenic (54a). Even one meal of these fish increases your cancer risk.

Our meat is just as bad. Testing of meat and poultry is done by the U. S. Department of Agriculture. They don't do it very well. A 1988 report from the USDA shows a litany of inspection errors: lost records, inadequate sampling, testing for only 20% of possible pesticides, and allowing meats to be sold that should have been impounded. In 28 cases reviewed in depth, 22 of the meat inspections were inadequate (55).

How can this happen in America? Many people still don't believe it. They think it is just another exaggerated fabrication of the media. Not so. It has been going on all the time. The Colgan Institute has monitored food pollution in America since 1980. The degree of pollution has not changed, only the degree of public outrage. We are realizing at last, that our food supply is seriously tainted.

On 26 May 1989, John Van de Camp, Attorney General of California, plus Public Citizen, the Natural Resources Defense Council and other environmental bodies, sued the EPA for it's failure to protect us from carcinogens. The lawsuit listed seven carcinogenic pesticides that are still in widespread use: benomyl, trifluralin, phosmet, chlordimeform, mancozeb, dichlorvos and dicofal. Anyone who reads the evidence presented with this lawsuit, and continues to buy regular dried figs, dates, raisins, barley, oats, wheat or rye, is just not serious about preventing cancer.

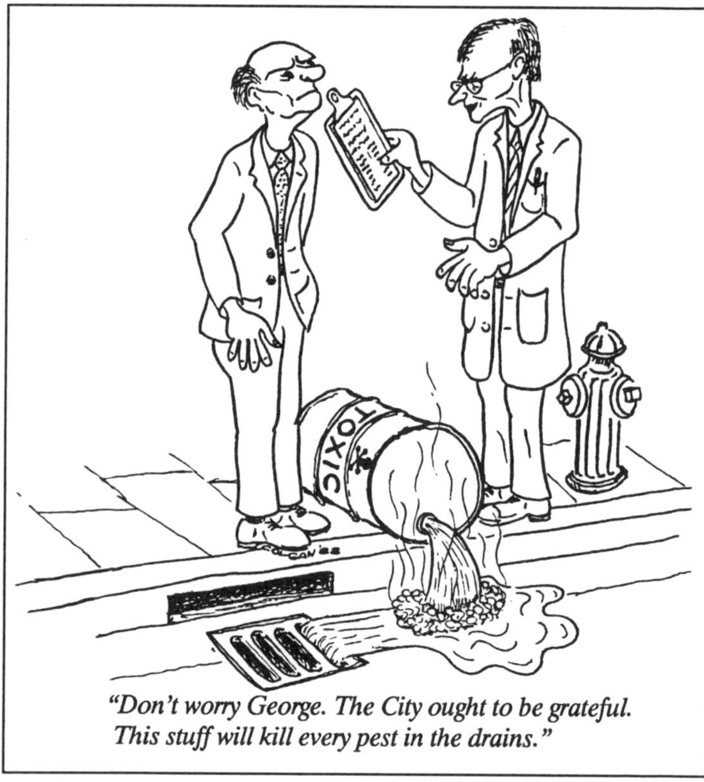

"Don't worry George. The City ought to be grateful. This stuff will kill every pest in the drains."

Protect Your Food

For produce, the solution is to buy American, and buy certified organic. Organically grown fruits and vegetables are on a roll. Twenty-six states now have organic food policies. Fifteen states have organic labeling laws. Seven more have or are planning state certification programs. Ring your state agency for information. Major supermarkets now stock organic produce, and produce that is certified free of pesticides. And health food markets are booming.

It is no longer a matter of going to the health food store to pick over a few pock-marked organic apples. America is starting to turn its agriculture back to the healthy condition of grandma's day. If the produce is not certified organic or certified pesticide free — don't buy it. The more you support the organic movement with your food dollars, the more you reduce the use of carcinogens. Voting with your pocketbook is a more powerful tool of democracy than any political party. Cast your vote against cancer.

If you have to make the transition more slowly, or you just cannot get organic produce where you live, Table 15 tells you how to treat regular produce. Exposure to pesticide residues can be reduced by 90%.

Table 15: How to Minimize Pesticide Residues in Produce

Produce	Treatment
Oranges, Bananas, Melons, and other peeling fruits	Peel and discard skin
Apples, Pears, Peaches, Apricots, Kiwis, Cucumbers, and Eggplant	Wash, peel and discard skin
Plums, Cherries, Grapes, Berry fruits, Celery, Corn, Broccoli, Cauliflower, Peppers, Green beans, Chinese peas	Buy only certified organic or certified pesticide free
Potatoes, Yams, Carrots	Soak and deeply peel
Peas	Discard pods
Dried beans	Soak. Protected by their original pods

Where's the Beef?

Your protein sources, fish, meat and dairy products, need careful selection. Avoid all fish from the Great Lakes. The EPA advises that all species are polluted with the carcinogens DDT, PCB's deildrin, aldrin, chlordane and toxaphene, plus numerous other banned substances. Pollution in the Great Lakes will continue for at least the next 50 years, because of run off of ground water from contaminated soil, and accumulation in the lake sediment of years of previous use of toxic substances.

Also heavily contaminated with DDT and PCB's are all species of fish and shellfish from the New York coast, the San Francisco Basin, the New Jersey coast, Puget Sound and the Boston Harbor area. Especially avoid the striped bass. In addition, ongoing studies by Dr Gary Wilkholm and Dr David Steinman with Loma Linda University show that fish from the Los Angeles coast now have some of the highest levels of DDT, and high levels of PCB's. Especially avoid mackerel, snapper, sole, halibut and butterfish.

Buy fish and shellfish from Australia, New Zealand and Scandinavia. They show only low levels of contamination. Fish from Alaska are clean also. The Exxon oil spill will not affect future supplies. If your store or restaurant does not know the origin of the fish, the offshore species are less contaminated, with the exception of swordfish. So choose cod, skipjack tuna, albacore, pollock, halibut and flounder. Freshwater brook trout and rainbow trout also have low levels of contamination, but don't eat the catfish.

Most beef is contaminated. Those delicious steaks at the supermarket are thankfully lower in fat these days, but they are all polluted with residues of hormones, antibiotics and other chemicals. Use of these chemicals, that speed growth and curb infections, is essential to compete in America's highly competitive mass meat market. With a little more concern for health, Europe recently rejected shipments of American beef, because pollutants exceeded their strict limits.

One recent example, reported by the Food and Drug Administration, is sulfamethazine. It is an effective drug against bacterial diseases in cattle and poultry. It is also a growth stimulant for hogs. At time of slaughter, levels of sulfamethazine in the meat must not exceed 100 parts per billion. The drug is completely illegal in milk.

The FDA reported in 1988 that one quarter of all milk samples were illegally contaminated with sulfamethazine. Figures for beef contamination are not available, but if there is that much in the milk, you can guess how bad the meat is. Over the last five years of FDA reports, 5-15% of all the pork tested showed illegal levels of the drug.

By the way, the FDA will tell you that sulfamethazine is a known carcinogen since 1988. Attempts have begun to limit its use. But it is cheap and effective, and well defended by the maker, American Cyanimid.

We looked at only one drug in meat and dairy products. FDA reports on numerous others are equally dismal. Ring the FDA and ask them. The warning is clear. If you want to avoid cancer, leave supermarket meats on the shelf.

Where's the **good** beef? A growing number of small ranches now raise beef that is certified free of all hormones and antibiotics, and is raised on chemical free grain. Best steaks you ever tasted. Two sources are Coleman's Natural Beef, P. O. Box 17045a, Denver, Colorado, 80217, and Maverick Ranch, 113 Livestock Exchange Building, Denver, Colorado, 80216. For a list of sources send SASE to Hormone Free Beef, 1501 16th Street, N.W., Washington, DC, 20036. These meats are also much lower in fats than regular beef: another plus in cancer prevention.

Drug-free poultry are now commonplace, even at the supermarket. Two brands are Foster Farms and Zacky Farms. Buy these in good health.

We don't have the space to cover prepared foods such as ketchup, peanut butter, jelly, spreads, fruit juice and sauces. But there are enough reasons given in previous sections to limit your use of these foods. Anyway, they are likely to be just as polluted as fresh foods.

I will give just one telling example. In early June 1989, national newspapers reported that Dennis Colleran, the president of Tree Top, the nation's largest processor of apples into juice and sauce, was forced to resign because of his vocal opposition to the use of Alar, and his refusal to buy Alar treated apples. Who is watching the store now?

Natural Food Carcinogens

Man-made carcinogens in food are not the only problem. Some foods carry potent carcinogens of their own. All peanut butter is contaminated with aflatoxin, the carcinogen that grows in mold in the peanuts. Amounts are usually tiny, and below the FDA limit, but present nonetheless. Dr Bruce Ames and colleagues rank a peanut butter sandwich as increasing cancer risk by 0.03% (55a).

Commercial mushrooms (*Agaricus bisporus*) naturally contain carcinogenic hydrazines. Their use carries a cancer risk of 0.1% (55a). Regular use of brown mustard carries a similar risk. It contains the natural carcinogen allyl isothiocyanate. The herbs tarragon, basil and fennel all contain the natural carcinogen estragole. Coffee, tea and red wine contain carcinogenic tannins. The umbelliferous vegetables, celery, parsnips and parsley all contain carcinogenic psoralens.

The herb comfrey is the worst. Though banned in other countries, it is still sold freely in America as a tea and in tablets. It contains the carcinogen symphytine and carries a completely unacceptable cancer risk of up to 6% (55a).

The best way around this problem is to limit your intake of these foods. Peanut butter is not a big worry, nor is the odd meal of mushrooms. I wouldn't eat comfrey, but it would probably take regular use for years to cause cancer. The healthy body has great defenses.

Food Pollution At Home

The final problem with food is what you do to it yourself. Storage and cooking habits can produce many carcinogens.

Fats and butters kept too long or kept for re-use after cooking will oxidize and produce carcinogens, including hydroperoxides, aldehydes and expoxides. Nuts and seeds left in the pantry can grow molds, almost impossible to see, but all containing the deadly carcinogen aflatoxin. And barbequing or open flame cooking of chicken, pork, beef and frankfurters produces the potent carcinogen benzopyrene, mainly in charred parts of the meat, and parts contaminated with smoke from burning fat (55b).

Lead is also a problem. Because of lead pollution, the bodies of most Americans carry 50 times the lead burden of their forefathers, leading to a variety of degenerative conditions. (55c, 55d). A lot of this lead comes from the leaded seams of cans. Dr D Mitchell tested 122 canned foods and beverages from food stores in New York. The average lead content was 80 mcg per pound of food (55e).

In the baby foods it was 100 mcg per pound. This level of lead pollution in regularly eaten foods is sufficient to cause brain damage, especially in an infant. Lead seepage into canned food accelerates when you open it. So never leave food in an open can. Better, don't use canned foods at all.

Chapter 17

Cancer on the Job

In 1979 the then Surgeon General reported that 2,300 chemicals are suspected carcinogens (10). Since then the number has escalated. Large numbers of Americans are polluted by these chemicals because of their job.

Job caused cancer is difficult to prove. Cancer is a degenerative disease that takes years to develop. You don't feel anything. You don't see anything. It grows insidiously inside you. When it finally becomes obvious, it is usually too late.

So workers go on using carcinogens and remain apparently healthy. Because they appear unaffected, health authorities are reluctant to believe the evidence that disease is silently happening. They are especially reluctant, if controlling the chemical will be costly for industry. Asbestos is the prime example. For years authorities denied that it was causing cancer. Now there are 12,000 lawsuits against the asbestos industry.

The Formaldehyde Debacle

Formaldehyde, a known carcinogen is a similar story. In 1982, Anne Gorsuch, then Administrator of the Environmental Protection Agency said that the problem of wide industrial use of formaldehyde was "**trivial**". Assistant Adminstrator John Todhunter agreed, and nothing was done. Industry lobbyists were happy to avoid the costs of making formaldehyde safe.

Then Gorsuch and Todhunter were ousted in the big EPA scandal. The Colgan Institute was among the many scientific organizations that protested to the new administration about formaldehyde. In 1984 the EPA agreed to re-open the file.

The EPA finally issued it's report on 16 April 1987, indicting formaldehyde as "a probable human carcinogen". Now, in November 1989, we are still waiting for most workers to be protected from it. There are over 780,000 workers in the garment industry exposed to formaldehyde, plus many hundreds of thousands in and around the plywood and particle board industries. In addition, formaldehyde is used in the manufacture of adhesives, detergents, dyes, fertilizers, insecticides, leathers, paints, paper and plastics. Workers in all these occupations are at risk.

In 1988 the Occupational Safety and Health Administration (OSHA) reduced the permissible exposure to formaldehyde by two-thirds, and required health warnings of possible cancer, and health monitoring of employees. Unfortunately, most cancers are neither found nor even suspected until they are well established. What is really required is regulation of the **emission** of formaldehyde into the air. We might get it by the turn of the century, but only if **you** demand it.

Plastics, Solvents and Gases

Even with well controlled chemicals, the occupational risk is not eliminated. Rubber vulcanization workers still have **10 times** the average risk of oesophageal cancer (50a). Workers in vinyl plastics industries have double the risk of lung cancer, and **two hundred times** greater risk of liver cancer, than the general population (10). Chances of a cure of either of these cancers is less than 10%. Rubber compounds and vinyl chloride exposure have been tightly controlled since the early 1970's, but the risk continues.

Other cancer hazards at work include coal tar, coke fumes from furnaces and ovens, coal dust, sand from sandblasting, and numerous chemicals in hair sprays, dyes and solvents. Methylene chloride, for example, is commonly used in hair sprays, as a solvent, as a flame retardent, and to decaffeinate coffee. It can cause cancer if inhaled. It still turns up despite a ban on it's use by the Food and Drug Administration.

Other inhaled chemicals that cause cancer are not banned. It is the height of irony that personnel in medical operating rooms, dedicated to saving lives, double their risk of cancer because of exposure to anaesthetic gases (51a).

Carcinogenic Metals

Metals on the job also pose a cancer risk. The worst risk industries are shown in Table 16. If you are serious about preventing cancer, then do not work with or near these metals. Further, do not buy a home on the down-wind side of these industries.

If you can't avoid a cancer risk occupation, then take all the precautions possible. Don't expect health authorities to protect you. You have to protect yourself. We have a rule in our lab that could benefit everyone in preventing cancer. *"Unless you can eat it, don't touch it or sniff it".*

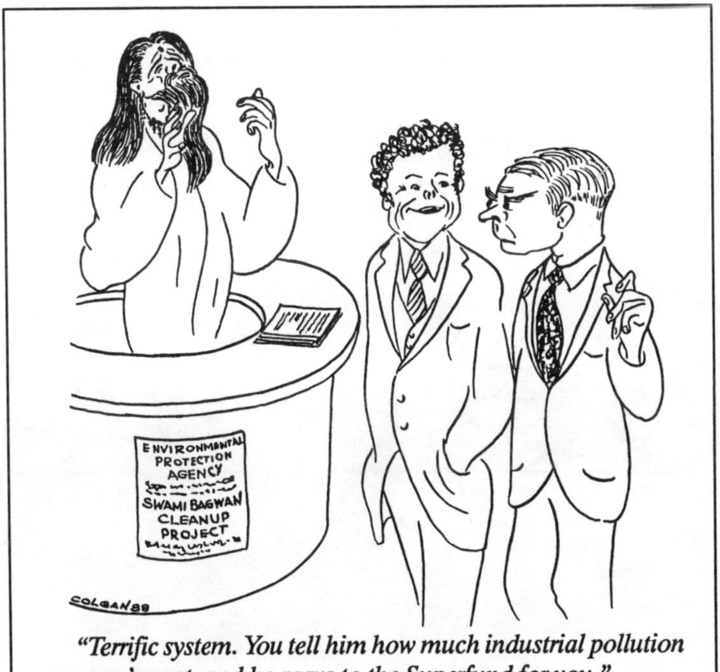

"Terrific system. You tell him how much industrial pollution you've got, and he prays to the Superfund for you."

Table 16: Occupational Exposure to Carcinogenic Metals

Metal	Occupation	Cancers Caused
Arsenic	Arsenic chemical plants	Lung
	Copper refineries	Skin
	Farm workers exposed to arsenic based pesticides	Liver
Cadmium	Cadmium refineries	Lung Prostate
Chromium	Chromium refineries	Gastrointestinal
	Chromate platers	Lung
	Chromate pigment workers	
Nickel	Nickel refineries	Lung Sinus Larynx, Kidney

Source: Sunderman (54)

Chapter 18

Keep Cancer Out Of The House

Your home may be hazardous to your health. Tobacco smoke is an obvious hazard, but, especially in new houses, formaldehyde leaks silently, undetected, from plywood, particle board, carpets, drapes and furniture. New materials can exude formaldehyde for four to eight years (57).

But the biggest carcinogenic hazard at home is likely to be radon gas. Radium is a naturally occurring component of soil and rock. Radon gas is its decay product. The gas seeps through the ground and through foundations, and accumulates in all homes. The better insulated the home, the more it accumulates.

Typical radon gas concentrations in houses range from 0.1 to 4.0 picocuries. But, in well sealed homes, concentrations can rise as high as 27 picocuries (56). To make sense of these numbers, beyond 4.0 picocuries is considered a cancer risk.

In May 1988, the EPA reported a three-year

study showing that radon gas in homes was causing 5,000 - 20,000 cases of lung cancer in America each year. In September 1988, the EPA and the Office of the Surgeon-General issued advisories, that every home in America be tested for radon gas. Most states are not yet set up to do this testing.

Don't wait until they are. You can obtain a test kit yourself for about $20. One source is Seventh Generation, 10 Farrel Street, Burlington, Vermont, 05403, (802)862-2999. They also sell home test kits for formaldehyde. If you find high levels of radon or formaldehyde, the solution is simple. Open the windows every day and let the wind blow it away.

In addition to radon and formaldehyde, homes are polluted by the release of chlorinated hydrocarbons, acetone, toluene, benzene and other carcinogens from paints, pesticides, cleaning products, air fresheners, hair sprays and cosmetics. The Consumer Product Safety Commission has identified over 100 chemicals in our homes that are linked to cancer. Even the permanent press finish on polyester/cotton bed linens exudes formaldehyde gas. Use pure cotton sheets instead. You will have better sleep and better health.

As with radon gas, the simple solution to indoor pollution is to open the windows a spell, every day. You can't do much about the outdoor air, but even in the worst polluted cities like New York and Los Angeles, outside air on most days is much less contaminated than the soup you are breathing inside. The EPA reports that inside air usually contains pollutants at two to five times outdoor levels.

The second solution is to buy natural products and fabrics, or those with certified non-toxic ingredients and finishes. Two good guides for getting the toxins out of your home are *House Dangerous*, by Ellen Greenfield (1989, Vintage Books) and *The Non-Toxic Home* by Debra Lynn Dadd (1986, JP Tarcher). They could save your health.

One other overlooked source of carcinogens in the home deserves note — your swimming pool. Because of the unregulated use of chlorine in home pools, the carcinogenic byproducts can reach dangerous levels. Children are especially at risk, because they are in the water longer and have less resistance to toxins of all kinds.

But you don't have to let your pool go green with algae and bacteria. That would be equally unsafe. Small water cleaning systems using no chlorine or similar chemicals, but instead using silver and copper ions in the filter system, have been used for years to clean water in laboratories. This method has now been expanded for use in larger bodies of water such as swimming pools.

The Colgan Institute has investigated five silver/copper systems now on the market. Only one really works well: Tarn Pure USA, phone (401)246-1246. In 1988 we built a 45 ft x 15 ft test pool, 3 ft to 7 ft deep, using the Tarn Pure, chemical free system to clean the water. Except when we had a burst pipe, in 15 months of operation, the system has kept the water free of algae and bacteria. It is like swimming in a mountain stream

— and, no carcinogens.

The biggest potential source of carcinogens at home lies in the garden, in unregulated use of the highly toxic chemicals sold to combat the vast array of insects, slugs and big bad bugs. Don't use these poisons. There are equally effective remedies that are virtually harmless to humans.

One example is *bacillus thuringiensis* that kills all kinds of caterpillers, corn borers, potato beetles and even gypsy moths. Another example is the green lacewing. This insect eats aphids, mealy bugs, scales, white fly and eggs of mites and other bugs. Then there is the ladybug, deadly on aphids, and decorative as well.

You can buy boxes of these and other beneficial insects, live, by mail. Distributed in your shrubbery they are very effective. For a poison-free garden, phone the Natural Gardening Research Center, P. O. Box 149, Summan, IN 47041, (812) 623-3800. The veggies taste better too.

Chapter 19

Ultra-Violet Causes Cancer

Dermatologists have warned us for decades that sunlight damages the skin. But most of us still refuse to give up the warm fuzzies of lying in the sun, and the golden glow that results.

Along with sunbathing, however, comes cancerous changes in the skin. Latest figures available from the National Cancer Institute show that in 1987, 526,000 Americans developed skin cancer. *The Journal of the American Medical Association* has just reported that squamous cell carcinoma has increased by 260% in men and 310% in women since 1960. Melanoma, the worst form of skin cancer, has increased 350% in men and 460% in women in the same period (58a).

One cause of these increases in skin cancer is the depletion of the stratospheric ozone layer by man-made chlorofluorocarbons (CFCs). CFCs were banned in aerosols in 1977, but they are still used widely as refrigerants and foaming agents in various industries (58b). On 3 October 1989, physicist Dr David Hofmann of the University of Wyoming, measured the ozone layer in Antarctica. This week he reported by telephone from New Zealand, that it was more depleted than in the early 1980s. The U. S. National Academy of Sciences estimates that every 1% reduction in the ozone layer will increase the incidence of different forms of skin cancer by 2 to 10 percent (58b).

Now, after years of squabbling, 23 countries have endorsed the Ozone Treaty, a plan to reduce CFC emissions by 50% by 1999. Meanwhile, millions of new cases of skin cancer will erupt caused by the increase in ultra-violet penetrating the damaged ozone layer (58).

You need not go outside to get skin cancer. Countless Americans use tanning beds. America boasts 18,000 tanning salons, all claiming to be absolutely safe if used as directed. Full of hyperbole and mendacity, a popular tanning chain pamphlet boasts: *"Our system uses only ultra-violet A (UVA), the good tanning wavelength, never ultra-violet B (UVB), the damaging, burning wavelength."*

Codswallop! Dr. John Epstein, dermatologist at the University of California, San Francisco, has shown that although UVA does not burn the skin surface so easily, it damages the underlying dermis. UVA is now considered the major cause of skin degeneration by sunlight. Also, exposure to UVA makes skin more prone to the cancer producing effects of UVB. All tanning beds cause skin damage, period.

You don't even have to visit a tanning bed. There is now very disturbing evidence that regular fluorescent lights, used in offices throughout the world, damage skin and may cause cancer.

Dr Valerie Beral and colleagues at the London School of Tropical Medicine, and at the University of Sydney in Australia, examined 274 women with malignant melanoma and compared them with 549 matched controls. With all other variables accounted for, fluorescent office lighting was associated with a 250% increase in risk of melanoma (58c).

The answer may lie in a crucial difference between the spectrum of office fluorescent lights and the spectrum of sunlight. Over millions of years of evolution, the human body learned to recognize and to develop mechanisms to protect itself from thousands of natural dangers including sunlight. It developed an inbuilt mechanism that responds to the precise mix of ultra-violet in sunlight by tanning and thickening the skin. This tanning response gives considerable protection against all skin damage, including skin cancer (58g).

But fluorescent light has a jagged emission spectrum. The body does not recognize it as dangerous, and does not protect itself by tanning, as the pasty faces of office workers attest. Yet fluorescent light **is** dangerous.Its jagged peaks of UVB can cause sunburn (58d, 58e), and it contains large amounts of UVA light of 315 - 400 nanometers, which has been shown to cause cancer in experimental animals (58h).

What's the solution? Except for those unfortunate few who cannot tan, it seems only sensible to use sunshine to get and maintain a **light** tan lifelong, to protect your skin from the unavoidable exposure to both indoor and outdoor ultra-violet light.

Sunscreens Help

If you must stay out in the sun, like mad dogs and Englishmen, then get the sunscreen habit. But it has to be the right sunscreen. For years most people have relied on creams with various Sun Protection Factor (SPF) ratings that contain para-amino-benzoic acid. That works fine against UVB, especially at SPF 15 and above. But it offers very little protection against UVA. To protect against UVA your sunscreen must also contain a benzone compound such as oxybenzone or benzophenone. One effective line of sun products that meets these criteria is Aloe Gator.

You cannot truly protect your skin, however, unless your diet contains sufficient of the nutrients that the skin uses to protect itself against cancer. The most important are: vitamin A, preferably eaten as beta carotene, vitamin E, vitamin B6, zinc and the mineral selenium. Note that, apart from zinc and vitamin B6, these are all from the antioxidants discussed in an earlier chapter. Skin damage from UV occurs mainly by oxidation.

This is not health food folklore. Recent studies at Cornell University for example, show that people with low dietary selenium have 440% increased risk of skin cancer (59). Also, mice given supplemental selenium show far less skin damage than controls (59).

Animal studies at the Xienta Institute for Skin Research (Bernville, PA) show that supplemental vitamin E also reduces sun damage. In another study, mice were given supplemental vitamin B6, then injected with live melanoma cells. The mice developed 62% fewer tumors than controls (60). The other nutrients, vitamin A and zinc are widely used in medicine to treat skin damage caused by their deficiency in diet. So with a little care to the skinside, and to what you put inside, you can still enjoy the sun in good health.

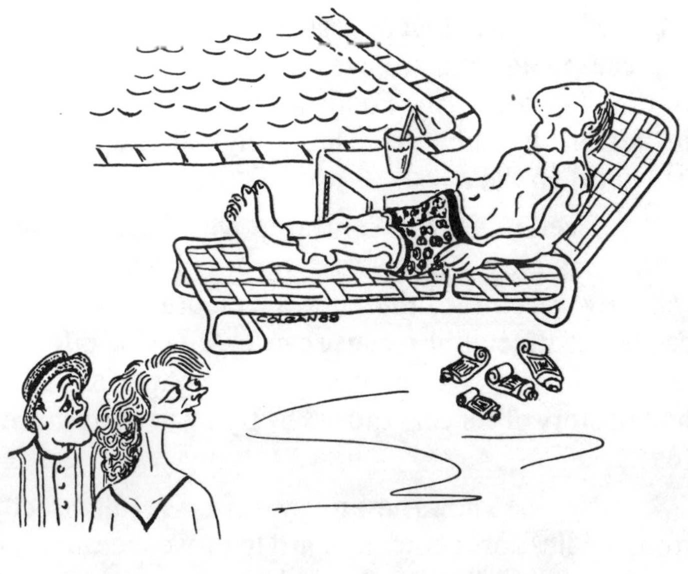

"Harry sometimes overdoes the sunscreen."

Chapter 20

Medication Causes Cancer

Anyone who reads the *Physician's Desk Reference,* cannot fail to be appalled at the number of medications listed that have strident warnings that they can cause cancer and have done so in experimental studies. Obviously, the Food and Drug Administration, in permitting their use, has weighed the benefits heavier than the risks.

Everything from contraceptive pills to common antibiotics have cancer risks recorded against them (68). Even some of the anti-cancer drugs and other cancer treatments also **cause** cancer, as a side effect of their use. Text books by physicians for physicians tell a horror story of cancers **caused** by trying to treat cancer (69).

No one knows how many cancers result directly from medication. Cases are hard to prove, because the physician's and the pharmaceutical company's insurers naturally defend themselves to the teeth! Official estimates from the National Cancer Institute put it at one in every 50 cancer deaths. **That is over 10,000 people a year.**

I will take just one example from the proven disasters of medical drugs. In the 1960's, the synthetic estrogen Diethylstilbestrol (DES) was an approved prescription drug to help prevent miscarriages. It worked, but in doing so, it also caused microscopic abnormalities to the womb, cervix and vagina of the growing female fetus. The babies appeared normal and grew into seemingly normal, healthy girls. But after puberty, some **fourteen to eighteen years after** their mothers' had taken the drug, 90% of these girls developed cancer of the vagina or reproductive system (69a, 69b).

It took researchers a long time to prove that DES was the cause of these cancers. It is banned now, but there are a lot more suspect drugs still out there. Both the FDA and the Surgeon General have warned repeatedly that overuse of prescribed medication is one of the biggest health hazards in America (69c, 69d, 69e).

Much of that medication is taken out of fear. Recently I advised a woman, made wretched by five prescribed drugs, to get a second opinion. She appeared in my office again sobbing — tears of joy. Her "heart condition" turned out be be a diagnostic error.

Use medications, even over-the-counter remedies, only when you have to. Take prescription drugs only after you have had the risks fully explained, and the necessity fully justified. It takes a hell of a justification to warrant swallowing carcinogenic medicine.

X-rays Cause Cancer

Even today, many Americans get routine X-rays for various occupations, for minor injuries and infections, and on admission to hospitals. Yet the Council of the American College of Radiology has recommended repeatedly that these practices be discontinued.

X-rays are carcinogenic, period. The evidence is irrefutable. Repeated X-rays cause breast cancer and increase the risk of leukemia in women (69f). In men, a lifetime exposure of 40 X-rays from chest to navel, increases risk of leukemia by **700%** (69g)!

Don't believe that those dinky little dental X-ray machines are safe either. They irradiate the brain as well as the teeth. There is hard evidence that repeated dental X-rays can cause brain cancer (70).

Rather than give more studies to convince you, let me quote from the conclusions of Dr John Gofman, Professor Emeritus of Medical Physics at the University of California, Berkely. In his 900 page textbook, *Radiation and Human Health*, he states,

> *...people, including physicians, have simply not realized that doses from medical diagnostic radiation are by no means low, even under the best of circumstances...and that the cancer risk of radiation is much more serious than they have been led to believe* (70).

Next time you are offered a routine X-ray say, "No thanks, trying to give them up."

Chapter 21

Exercise Prevents Cancer

The National Cancer Institute fails to recommend regular exercise, despite mounting evidence that particular forms of exercise are cancer preventative.

People who exercise to gain a high level of lean tissue (muscle) are on the right track. As I discussed earlier, animal and human studies indicate that being super lean is one of the strongest cancer preventatives. So particular types of exercise that get you the highest ratio of lean weight to fat weight, are the best sports to prevent cancer. The most effective of these is weight training.

Building muscle is not the only cancer preventative aspect of exercise. Most cancers are partly caused by degeneration of the body with age, until the influence of one or other carcinogens overcomes its weakened defenses. Remember, no one dies of old age. We die of disease. And after heart disease, cancer is the biggest disease risk of aging.

Weight training exercise can at least slow down this age degeneration. Writing in the *Journal of the*

American Medical Association, Dr Walter Bortz of the Department of Medicine of the Palo Alto Medical Clinic in California, reviewed over 100 studies which indicated that many degenerative changes usually attributed to aging, are in fact caused by lack of regular exercise (61).

Jogging or running by itself will not do, because it does not maintain upper body muscle. Swimming will not do, because it does not stop deposition of bodyfat, nor maintain bone mass. Tennis will not do, because it does not maintain muscle mass or cardiovascular fitness.

Weight training plus an aerobic sport can prevent or slow down, loss of strength, loss of bone mass, loss of muscle mass, degeneration of glucose tolerance, loss of cardiovascular fitness, decline of hormone levels, and decline of the immune system (61). All these degenerative changes weaken you and make you prey to cancer.

A minimum exercise program that could be considered cancer preventative might be as follows. REMEMBER, don't start any exercise program without being cleared by your physician.

For aerobic exercises, do **one** of the following:

	# of days per week	minutes per day
Walking	3 - 4	30 - 40
Cycling	3 - 4	30 - 40
Jogging	3 - 4	20 - 30
Rowing	3 - 4	20 - 30
Swimming	3 - 4	30 - 40

To optimize the ratio of lean tissue to fatty tissue use a

specific weight training program. The minimum program is 3 workouts per week of about 45 minutes. Each workout should include 15 - 20 exercises. All three workouts together should cover all the major muscles of the body.

For detailed information on the type of lifelong exercise program most effective in preventing degeneration, contact the Colgan Institute (619) 632-7722. You don't have to kill yourself. For greatest use of bodyfat for fuel, aerobic exercise should be of moderate intensity. Recent studies show that aerobic exercise at 40% of maximum effort is the most effective (61a). So run for your life, but run easy.

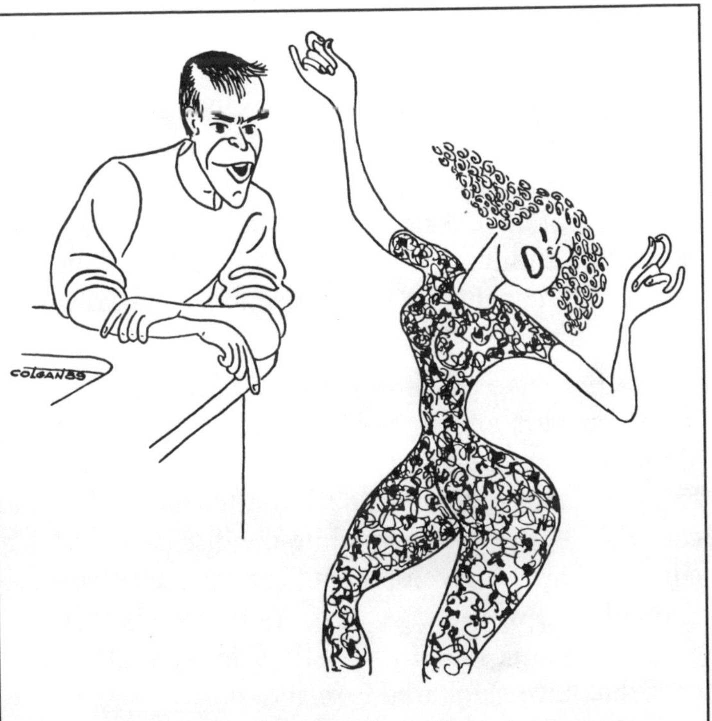

"Those hi-impact aerobics did lower your weight Alice, but I don't think you lost any."

Chapter 22

Screening Helps

Screening for cancer helps - sometimes. We are not talking about the ubiquitous annual physical. Annual medical examinations are a failure at detecting disease. For example, an extensive study for the Kaiser Health Plan tested 10,000 people aged 35-54. Five thousand were given frequent medical examinations and 5,000 were left alone. Over seven years, there was no difference between the groups in the incidence of disease, nor in the death rate (62). After reviewing numerous similar studies at the Colgan Institute, we reluctantly concluded that the annual checkup is a waste of time.

Effective cancer screens are specific tests such as Pap smears and sigmoidoscopy. Pap smears work. This test, named for its inventor, Dr. George Papanicolaou, gives women a better chance of beating cancer by early detection, while the disease is still in a curable stage of development. The test, which can be applied to a wide range of cancers, not just cervical cancer, examines bodily secretions looking for cancer cells that have exfoliated from a tumor.

The American Cancer Society periodically

changes its mind about whether or not annual Pap tests are necessary. Probably the best advice is to have one each three years after having two successive annual tests with a clean result. Localized cancers detectable by Pap smears are uncommon (less than 20,000 cases a year), slow growing, and almost always curable.

Sigmoidoscopy tests also work.They detect colorectal cancer, the third most common cancer in America. There is a popular misconception that it occurs mainly in men. In fact, colorectal cancer occurs equally in both sexes. The test is very effective in detecting this cancer while there is still a chance of a cure. Prior to 50 years of age, for healthy people with no family history of colorectal cancer, a test every 5-10 years is probably sufficient. Thereafter, every three years is sensible.

Unlike sigmoidoscopy, stool sample tests for colorectal cancer are not effective. They often give high levels of false results (64). The same goes for breast self-examination in women. It is not as useful as the health media would have you believe. It takes 10-20 years for most breast tumors to reach a size that can be felt in this way. Suspicious lumps should always be reported to your physician, but most detective work of this kind is likely to be unsuccessful (65, 66, 67). It may then become counter-productive by providing a crutch of false confidence.

Mammography for breast cancer is more effective, and can detect a breast cancer long before it can be felt by hand. On 27 June 1989, eleven U. S. Health authorities, including the National Cancer Institute, the American Medical Association and the American Cancer Society, finally came to a concensus about mammography. All women are now recommended to have mammograms every two years from age 40 to 49, and annually thereafter. New, much lower power X-rays, have made the procedure safer. Taking the X-ray is still a risk/benefit decision, but the research shows that early detected breast cancer can be cured. So it seems a sensible precaution.

Testicular examination in men can also provide some early detection. But self-examination is tricky. A lot of men have lived in terror for months, after feeling a suspicious lump. When they finally get the courage to go to their physician, it turns out to be the very common, but harmless, testicular cyst. Better to let the professional do it in the first place, and save yourself a lot of grief.

The classic case of failure of early detection is that of lung cancer. In 1979 the then Surgeon-General stated in his *Report On Health Promotion and Disease Prevention* ,

> *Early identification techniques such as chest X-rays and sputum examinations generally do not discover lung cancer before it has spread.* (p65)

So use cancer screening judiciously, but don't rely on it. Don't think you can neglect nutrition and exercise because you come out clean on an annual cancer screen.

Chapter 23

The Anti-cancer Lifestyle

Your body is a hollow tube. From mouth to anus is one continuous tunnel. Your lungs, a side chamber off the tunnel, are stuffed with delicate tissues exposed to the air you breathe. Like your skin, the surface of your internal tunnel is exposed to the environment, the air, water and food you take in, and the toxins and carcinogens they contain.

Over 90% of all cancers occur on these external and internal exposed surfaces. Less than 10% of cancers occur within the body, in tissues not exposed to the environment, compelling evidence that the cause of most cancers lies in our environment.

Despite the mountain of regulatory controls, we have all seen how environmental poisons are increasing. It is not surprising then, that the incidence of cancer is increasing also.

A new two-year study by the Congressional Office of Technology Assessment (OTA) was released to Congress on 19 October 1989. Previous estimates counted 1,200 toxic waste sites nationwide, that are leaching large amounts of carcinogenic chemicals into surrounding soils. These chemicals can spread for hundreds of miles through the ground-water, to contaminate your soil, your farm,and the meat and produce it grows.

The new study shows that the problem is much worse than we thought. The OTA has uncovered evidence that the number of leaking toxic waste sites is not 1,200, but more than 10,000! It also showed that the Superfund, a $10.1 billion cleanup effort created in 1980, has been almost totally ineffective. Our poisoned environment is here to stay—at least in our lifetimes.

As this greater environmental attack burdens our immune systems every day, reducing their capacity to deal with disease, it is not surprising either, that our bodies have less chance of curing cancer than they did a quarter century ago. The only real defense is to protect your exposed body surfaces, and strengthen your immune defenses, so as to prevent cancer from becoming established.

I have reviewed some of the pertinent studies that show how particular nutrition, exercise and lifestyle practices can remove most risks of cancer from your life. They are summarized in Table 17. In essence they are the practices that reduce the risks of all degenerative diseases. For cancer is a degenerative disease, silently established, slow and silent to grow, taking perhaps 20 years to show, only **after** it has ravaged the body.

Medicine cannot detect the start of degenerative disease. Nor can it cure the final stages. The billions spent since the 60s in America's "war on cancer," have been wasted for almost naught. There will never be a"magic bullet" against cancer to claim Armand Hammer's $1,000,000 prize. The only way is **host resistance**. You have to protect yourself.

Do not fear cancer. Instead, respond aggressively to the added cancer burden of our ever more poisoned world. As Dr Lewis Thomas, President of the Sloan Kettering Cancer Hospital in New York reminds us, the human body is incredibly tough. Given the right nutrition, exercise and lifestyle, it will reject cancer every day for a lifetime. Put your body in that state and join me for the 21st century of human progress.

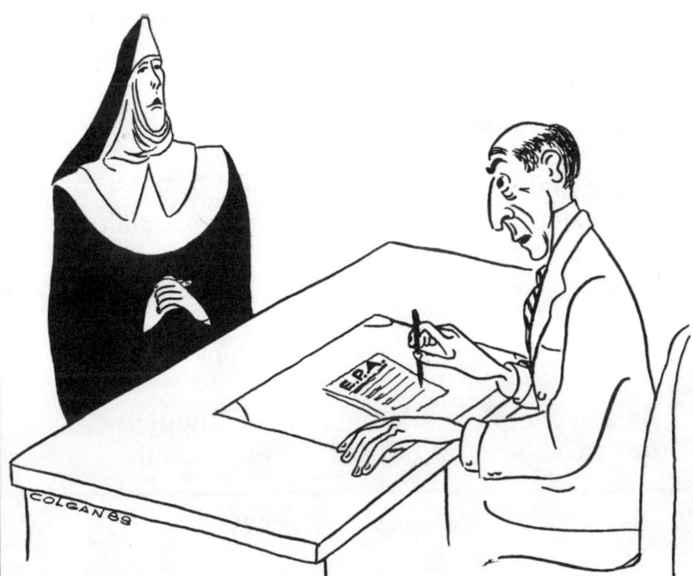

"Let me get this straight. Beelzebub has filed a complaint with the Man Upstairs that we are polluting the fiery furnace?"

TABLE 17: The Cancer Prevention Lifestyle*

1. Don't smoke.
   Don't permit others to puff their smoke about you.

2. Drink alcohol moderately if at all.
   (Maximum: 2 beers or 2 singles of liquor or 2 glasses of wine per day).

3. Maintain low bodyfat.
   (Men 8-15%. Women 14-21%).

4. Eat a moderate calorie diet.

5. Eat a low-fat diet.
   (Maximum: 25% of daily calories as fat).

6. Eat a high fiber diet.
   (40-60 grams a day).

7. Eat a high level of vegetables and fruits.
   (Use only fresh produce, certified organic or certified pesticide free).

8. Eat a nutrient dense diet.
   (Avoid refined, canned, preserved and processed foods).

9. Take a complete vitamin/mineral supplement.
   (Minimum: Twice the USRDA of every nutrient).

Continued on Page 125

Table 17: Continued

10. Take a high level of antioxidants.
11. Ensure intake of essential fatty acids.
    (Linoleic acid and linolenic acid).
12. Avoid cancer risk occupations.
13. Drink and cook with properly purified water.
14. Protect yourself from food pollution.
15. Free your home of carcinogens.
16. Protect your skin from ultra-violet light.
17. Exercise regularly by weight training plus an aerobic sport.
18. Take the cancer screens advised.
19. Avoid all medications and X-rays except when essential to treatment of disease.

***This list is compiled from reviews of the medical and scientific evidence. It is presented for information purposes only.**

References

1. Bailor, J. C., Smith, E. M., *New England J Med*, 1986, *314*, 1226.
2. *Nutrition and Fitness* Vol I to VIII. San Diego: The Colgan Institute, 1982-1989.
3. Culliton, B. J., *Science*, 1987, *236*, 380.
4. Personal communication. Figures obtained by the Colgan Institute from the National Cancer Institute, December 1988.
5. National Cancer Institute, *Cancer Prevention*, NIH Publication No 84-2671, Washington DC, Department of Health and Human Services, 1984.

5a. Yu, B.P., et al. *J Gerontology*, 1982, *37*, 130.

5b. Roe, F. J. *Nature*, 1983, *303*, 657.

6. *The 1988 Surgeon General's Report on Nutrition and Health.* Publication No PHS 88-50210, Washington DC: Department of Health and Human Services, 1988.
7. Editorial, Screening for Alcoholism, *Lancet*, 1980, *2*, 1117.
8. Horrobin, D. F., *Medical Hypotheses,* 1980, *6*, 929.
9. *The Harvard Medical School Health Letter*, 1981, *7*, 2.
10. The Surgeon General. *Healthy People: The Surgeon General's Report on Health Promotion and Disease Prevention.* DHEW Publications Nos 79-55071 and 79-55071A, Washington DC: DHEW 1979.

10a. Correa, P., el al, *Lancet*, 1983, *10 September*, 595.

10b. Hirayama, T., *Brit Med J*, 1981, *282*, 183.

10c. Trichopoulos, D., et al, *Int J Cancer*, 1981, *27*, 1.

11. American Cancer Society. *Cancer Prevention Study*, 1959-1979, New York: American Cancer Society, 1980.
12. Abraham, S., Johnson, C. L., *Vital and Health Statistics of the National Center for Health Statistics*, DHEW Publication No. 51, Hyattsville, MD, 1979.
13. Schwartz, R. S., Brunzell, J. D., *J Clin Invest*, 1981, *67*, 1425.
14. Elliot, D. L., et al, *Amer J Clin Nutr*, 1989, *49*, 93.
15. Fisher, M., La Chance, P., *J Amer Dietetic Assoc*, 1985, *85*, 112.
16. *Amer J Public Health*, 1988, Sept/Oct.
17. *Amer J Clin Nutr*, 1985, *41*, 1177.

18. Tipton, H., Stewart, P. L., in Hemphill, D.D. (Ed). *Trace Substances in Environmental Health*, Columbia Md: University of Missouri Press, 1985.
19. Felig, L., *Clinical Physiology*, 1984, *4*, 267.
20. Storlien, L. H., *Science*, 1987, *237*, 885.
21. Bielinski, R. *Amer J Clin Nutr*, 1985, July.
22. Mc Cay, C. M., *J Nutr*, 1939, *18*, 1.
23. Ross, M. H., in Winick, M. (Ed). *Nutrition and Aging*, New York: Wiley, 1976.
24. Weindruch, R., Walford, R., *Science*, 1982, *215*, 1415.
24a. Cheney, K. E., et al, *Exp Gerontol*, 1980, *15*, 237
24b. Ross, M. H., Bras, G., *Journal of the National Cancer Institute*, 1971, *47*, 1095
25. Bull, A. W., et al, *Cancer Res*, 1979, *39*, 4956.
26. *Diet, Nutrition and Cancer*, Washington, DC: National Academy Press, 1982, 5-20.
27. Silverman, J. J., *Amer Med Assoc*, 1981, *179*, 1404.
28. Lin, K., et al, *Lancet*, 1979, *2*, 782.
29. Waterhouse, J., et al, *Cancer Res*, Vol. 3, Lyon: WHO International Agency for Research on Cancer, 1976.
30. Glober, G. A., et al, *Lancet*, 1977, *2*, 110.
30a. Story, J. A., Kritchevsky, D., *J Nutr*, 1976, *106*, 1292.
30b. Reddy, B. S., Wynder, E. L., *J Nat Cancer Inst*, 1973, *50*, 1437.
31. Burkitt, D. P., *Lancet*, 1972, 2, 1408.
31a. De Cosse, J., et al, *J Nat Cancer Inst*, 1989, September
32. Wattenberg, L. W., in Arnott, M. S., et al, (Eds). *Molecular Interraltions of Nutrition and Cancer*, New York: Raven Press, 1982, 43.
33. Wattenberg, L.W., et al, *Cancer Res*, 1980, *40*, 2820.
34. Pantuck, E. J ., et a, *Clin Pharmacol Ther*, 1979, *25*, 88.
35. Wattenberg, L. W., Loub, W. D., *Cancer Res*, 1978, *38*, 1410.
36. Wattenberg, L. W., Leong, J. L., *Cancer Res*, 1970, *30*, 1922.
37. Wattenberg, L. W., et al, *J Nat Cancer Inst.*, 1979, *62*, 1103.
38. Bock, G., et al, *Amer J Epidemiol*, 1988, *127*, 297.
38a. Wohl, M. G., Goodheart, R.S., (eds) *Modern Nutrition in Health and Disease*, 3rd Edition, Philadelphia: Lea & Febiger, 1964.
38b. Williams, R. J. in Hawkins, D., Pauling, L., (Eds) *Orthomolecular Psychiatry*, San Francisco: WH Freeman, 1973, 316.

38c. Williams, R. J., Pelton, R.B., *Proc Nat Acad Sci USA*, 1966, *55*, 126.
39. *First Health and Nutrition Examination Survey United States* 1971-1972, Rockville, MD: DHEW Publications 76-1219-1, 1976.
39a. Nationwide Food Consumption Survey Preliminary Report No. 2, Washington DC: USDA, 1980.
39b. US Department of Agriculture, *Food Technology*, 1981, *35*, 9.
39c. *American J Clin Nutr*, 1985, *41*, 1177.
39d. *Recommended Dietary Allowances, 9th Edition*, Washington, DC: National Academy of Science, 1980.
39e. Holden, J. M., Wolf, W. R., Mertz, W., *J Am Diet Assoc.*, 1979, *75*, 23.
40. Colgan, M., *Your Personal Vitamin Profile*, New York: Morrow, 1982.
41. Colgan, M., in Katch, F. (Ed) *Sport Health and Nutrition*, Champaign, Ill: Human Kinetics, 1986, 21.
41a. Burkitt, D., Trowell, H. C., *Western Diseases: Their Emergence and Prevention*, Cambridge, Mass: Harvard University Press, 1981.
41b. American Medical Association Council on Food and Nutrition, *Nutrients In Processed Foods*, Acton, Mass: Publishing Sciences Group, 1974.
41c. Schroeder, H. A., *Am J Clin Nutr*, 1971, *24*, 562.
42. Ames, B., *Science*, 1983, *221*, 1256.
43. Cameron, E., Pauling, L., *Cancer and Vitamin C*, New York: Warner Books, 1981.
44. Bjelke, E., Scand, J., *Gastroenterology*, 1974, *9*, Supplement 31.
45. Wagner, D., *Cancer Res*, 1985, *45*, 6519.
45a. Benedict, W. F., Jones, P. A., In Arnott, M.S., et al (Eds) *Molecular Interrelations of Nutrition and Cancer*, New York: Ravey Press, 1982, 351.
46. Knekt, P., et al, *Amer J Epidemiol*, 1988, *127*, 28.
46a. Knekt, P., *Internal J Epicem*, 1988, *17*, 281.
46b. Horvath, P. M., Ip, C., *Cancer Res*, 1983, *43*, 5335.
46c. Menkes, M. S., *New Eng J Med*, 1986, *315*, 1250.
46d. Watson, R. R., Leonard, T. K., *J Am Diet Assoc*, 1986, *86*, 505.
47. Kummet, T., Meyskins, F., *Seminars in Oncology*, 1983, *10*, 281.
48. Menkes, M. S., et al, *New England J Med*, 1986, *315*, 1250.
48a. Hirayama, T., *Nutr Cancer*, 1979, *1*, 67.

48b. Stich, H. F., et al, *Lancet*, 1984, *1*, 1204.
48c. Ames, B. N., *Science*, 1983, *221*, 1256.
48d. Knekt, P., et al, 4th International Symposium of Selenium, Tubingen, Germany, July, 1988. (Abstract)
48e. Reinhold, U., et al, 4th International Symposium on Selenium, Tubingen, Germany, July, 1988. (Abstract)
48f. *Recommended Dietary Allowances, 9th Edition*, Washington, DC, 1980.
48g. Wartholm, M., et al, *Biochem Biophys Res Comm*, 1981, *98*, 512.
48h. Richie, J. P., *Gerontologist*, 1983, *23*, 76.
48j. Schneider, D., et al, *Fed Proc Fed Am Soc Exp Biol*, 1982, *41*, 3570.
48k. Weber, H., et al, *Arch Gerontol Geriat*, 1982, *1*, 299.
48l. Novi, A. M., *Science*, 1981, *242*, 541.
48m. *Biomedical and Clinical Aspects of CoEnzyme Q Vols 1 - 4*, New York: Elsevier, 1977-1984.
49. Coldetz, A., et al, *Amer J Clin Nutr*, 1985, *41*, 32.
49a. Tengerdy, R. P., et al, *Infect Immun*, 1972, *5*, 987.
49b. Henzerling, R. H., et al, *Infect Immun*, 1974, *10*, 1292.
49c. Spallholtz, J. E., et al, *Proc Soc Exp Biol Med*, 1973, *143*, 685.
49d. Tengerdy, R. P., in Phillips, M., Baetz, A., (Eds) *Advances in Exper Med and Biol Diet and Resistance to Disease, Vol 135*, New York: Plenum, 1981, 40.
49e. Basten, A., Mitchell, J. in Nelson, D. S. (Ed), *Immunobiology of the Macrophage*, New York: Academic Press, 1976, 43.
49f. Good, R. A., et al, in Susskind, R. M. (Ed) *Malnutrition and the Immune Response*, New York: Raven Press, 1977, 169.
49g. Homan-Muller, J. W., et al, *J Lab Clin Med*, 1975, *85*, 198.
49h. McCord, J. M., *Science*, 1974, *185*, 529.
49j. Schrauzer, G. N., *Ann Clin Lab Sci*, 1974, *4*, 441.
49k. Kiremidjian-Schumacher, L., Stotzy, G., *Environ Res*, 1987, *42*, 277.
49l. Harman, D., et al, *J Am Geriat Soc*, 1977, *9*, 400.
49m. Bliznakov, E., *Biomedical and Clinical Aspects of CoEnzyme Q*, New York: Elsevier, 1977.
50. Erasmus, U., *Fats and Oils*, Vancouver: Alive Books, 1986.
50a. Norell, S., et al, *Lancet*, 1983, *1*, 462.
51. Horrobin, D. F., (Ed) *Clinical Uses of Essential Fatty Acids*, London: Eden Press, 1982.

51a. *Anaesthesiology*, 1974, *41*, 321.
51b. Dippenaar, N., et al, *S A Med J*, 1982, *82*, 505.
51c. Tanure, R., et al, *Nutrition and Cancer*, 1988, *11*, 215.
51d. Campbell, T. C., *J Nat Cancer Inst*, 1989, 7 June.
52. *Nutrition News*, 1987, 6, *3*, 14.
53. Conn, P., *Not a Drop to Drink*, Cleveland, TN: Carroll Printing Co., 1980.
54. Sunderman, F. W., *Biol and Trace Element Res*, 1979, *1*, 63.
54a. Foran, J. A., *Amer J Public Health*, 1989, March.
55. USDA FSIS Monitoring and Controlling Pesticide Residues in Domestic Meat and Poultry Products. Washington, DC, 1988.
55a. Ames, B., et al, *Science*, 1987, *236*, 271.
55b. Larsson, B. K., et al, *J Agric Food Chem*, 1983, *31*, 867.
55c. Needleman, H., et al, *N Eng J Med*, 1979, *300*, 689.
55d. Waldron, H., Stofen D., *Subclinical Lead Poisoning*, New York: Academic Press, 19784.
55e. Mitchell, D. G., Aldous, K. M., *Environ Health Pespect*, 1974, 7, 59.
56. Nero, A. V., Lawrence Berkelley Laboratory Publications, LBL-10525, 1981, August.
57. Spengler, J. D., Sexton, K., *Science*, 1983, *221*, 9.
58. *Science*, 1986, *234*, 927.
58a. *J Amer Med Assoc*, 1989, 20 October.
58b. *Cancer and Effects of Stratospheric Ozone Reduction: An Update*, Washington, DC: National Academy Press, 1982.
58c. Beral, V., et al, *Lancet*, 1982, *7 August*, 290.
58d. Jewess, B. W., *Soc Photo-optical Instrumentation*, 1981, *262*, 55.
58e. Brown, S., et al, *Brit J Dermatol*, 1969, *81*, 420.
58f. Beral, V., Robinson, N., *Brit J Cancer*, 1981, *44*, 886.
58g. Robertson, D. F., *Med J Australia*, 1968, *2*, 1123.
58h. Magnus, I. A., Young, A. R., *Proc Internat Psoralens SIR*, Paris: Pergamon Press, 1981.
59. Thorling, E. B., *Acta Pathol Microbiol Immunol Scand*, 1983, *91A*, 81.
60. DiSorbo, D., *Nutrition and Cancer*, 1985, *7*, 43.
61. Bortz, W., *J Amer Med Assoc*, 1982, *248*, 1203.
61a. Ahlborg, G., Felig, P., *J Appl Physiol*, 1976, *41*, 683.
62. *Consumer Reports*, 1980, *October*, 601.

63. American Society for Gastrointestinal Endoscopy. *J Amer Med Assoc*, 23 Jan 1989.
64. Knight, K., *J Amer Med Assoc*, 23 Jan 1989.
65. Sutherland, R., *Cancer: The Significance of Delay*, London: Butterworth, 1960.
66. Atkins, J., *Brit Med J*, 1972, *2*, 423.
67. Byar, D. P., *J Urology*, 1972, *108*, 908.
68. *AMA Drug Evaluations, 4th Edition*, Littleton, Mass.: American Medical Association, 1980.
69. Schmal, D., et al, *Iatrogenic Cacinogenesis*, New York: Springer Verlag, 1977.
69a. American Medical Association, *AMA Drug Evaluations, 4th Edition*, Littleton, Mass: AMA, 1980, 678.
69b. Bichler, J., *DES Daughter*, New York: Avon, 1981.
69c. *Science*, 1973, *180*, 1038.
69d. Wade, N., *Science*, 1973, *179*, 775.
69e. The Surgeon General, *Healthy People: The Surgeon General's Report on Health Promotion and Disease Prevention,* Washington: DHEW, 1979, PUB. Nos. 7955071, 7955071A.
69f. Gofman, J. W., *Radiation and Human Health*, San Francisco: Sierra Book Club, 1981.
69g. Gibson, R., et al, *J Nat Cancer Inst*, 1972, *48*, 301.
70. Gofman, J. W., *Radiation and Human Health*, San Francisco: Sierra Club Books, 1981.

Index

A

Acids:,
  docosahoxanoic, 80
  eicosapentanoic, 80
  trans fatty, 80
  cis, 80
Aging and:
  calories, 27
  l-glutathione, 70, 71
Alar, 11, 88, 95
Alcohol, 17
  chemicals in 17, 18
  excess, 18
  safe limit, 18
Alcohol and
  liver cancer, 17
  mouth cancer, 17
  oesophagus cancer, 17
  throat cancer, 17
Alcoholics, 18
Alexander Medical Foundation, 70
Aloe Gator Sunscreen, 110
American Cancer Society, 11, 19, 47, 118, 120
American College of Radiology, 114
American Cyanimid, 94
American Medical Association, 57, 120
Ames, Bruce 11, 64, 69, 96
Annual physical, 118
Antioxidants: 63
  beta carotene 63, 67
  coenzyme q10, 63
  l-glutathione, 63
  selenium, 63
  vitamin A, 63, 67
  vitamin C, 63, 64
  vitamin E, 63, 66
Antioxidants, amount required, 78
Antioxidants, increasing immune strength, 75
Antioxidants and:
  immune system, 74-77
  immunity, 74 - 77
  reduced cancer, 76
Athletic Performance,
  effect of multi-nutrient supplementation on, 55
Atkins Diet, 22
Attorney General of California, 5

B

Bailor, John, 2, 3
Beef:
  Colman's, 95
  contaminated, 94
  good, 95
  Maverick Ranch, 95
Benedict, William, 65
Benzophenone, 110
Beral, Valerie, 109
Berg, Benjamin, 27
Beta carotene & reduced cancer, 67, 68
Beverly Hills Diet, 22
Bjelke, E., 64
Bliznakov, Emile, 73
Block, Gladys, 46
Bloody rout, 3, 4
Bodyfat and:
  complex carbohydrates, 25
  sugar, 25
Bodyfat:
  rate to lose, 25
  rules for losing, 25-26
Bortz, Walter, 116
Bras, G, 28

Bread:
- enriched and cancer, 50
- white and metabolism, 49, 50
- white and cancer, 49, 50
- whole grain, 51

Breast cancer, 3, 4

Breast cancer:
- and fat, 30
- death rate, 4
- detection, 4
- improvement, 4

Breast, self examination, 119

Brynner, Yul, 15

Bull, A.W., 30

Burkitt, Dennis, 42

C

Calories, 25

Calories and:
- cancer, 27
- aging, 27

Cameron, Ewan, 64

Campbell, Colin, 81

Cancer and:
- calories, 27
- diethylstilbestrol, 113
- enriched bread, 50
- white bread, 49, 50

Cancer:
- causes, 11, 13
- cure, 3
- death rate 2, 3, 6
- deaths in America, 3
- degenerative disease, 9
- incidence, 6, 28
- mortality, 7
- new cases 1989, 6
- prevention 8, 11, 12
- risk factors, 10, 13
- screens, 118
- statistics update, 6
- treatment, 8

Cancer, types of:
- colorectal, 40
- liver, 100

Cancer, types of (con't)
- lung, 100

Cancer, reduced and:
- antioxidants, 76
- beta carotene, 67, 68
- coenzyme Q10, 73
- essential fatty acids, 81
- l-glutathione, 70, 71
- selenium, 69
- vitamin C, 64
- vitamin E, 66

Cancer prevention lifestyle, 124-125

Canned food, lead in, 97

Carcinogenic vegetables, 96

Carcinogens:
- at home, 103
- in gardens, 106
- in swimming pools, 105
- industrial, 98
- in metals, 101, 102
- natural, 96

Carcinoma, squamous cell, 107

Cellulose triacetete membrane, 86

Chest X-rays, 120

Chlorine, 11

Chlorofluorocarbons, 107,

Chromium and fat loss, 26

Cis fatty acids, 80

Coenzyme Q10, 73

Coenzyme Q10, amount required, 73

Coenzyme Q10 and reduced cancer, 73

Coffee, 96, 100

Cold pressed oils, 79, 80

Coleman's Beef, 95

Colgan Institute, 2, 11, 18, 24, 42, 46, 64, 69, 85, 86, 89, 117

Colleran, Dennis, 95

Colon cancer and fat, 30

Colorado State Unvirsity, 74

Colorectal cancer, 40

Colorectal cancer and fiber, 41

Comfrey, 96

Complex carbohydrates and bodyfat, 25
Congressional Office of Technology Assessment (COA), 121
Cooking oils, 81, 82, 83
Corn oil, 81
Cornell University, 81
Correa, Pelayo, 14

D

Dadd, Debra Lynn, 105
DeCosse, Jerome, 41
Dental X-rays, 120
Department of Public Health, 84
DeVita, Vincent, 3, 4
Diet, high fiber, 40
Dietary regain of fat 21, 24
Diethylstilbestrol (DES) and cancer, 113
Dieting, 20, 21
Dieting and metabolic rate, 21
Diets and:
  bodyfat, 20, 21
  fiber, 22
  Dieting, 20, 21
  the RDAs, 22
Diets:
  dangerous, 22
  medical, 24
  popular, 23
Dipenaar, Nola, 81
Docosahexanoic acid, 80
Doll, Richard, 11

E

Eicosapentanoic acid, 80
Elliot, Diane, 21
Environmental pollution, 5
Environmental Protection Agency (EPA), 5, 88, 99
Environmental Protection Agency, lawsuit against 89-90
Epstein, John, 108
Essential fatty acids, 79-83
Essential fatty acids & reduced cancer, 81
Essential fatty acids:
  cold pressed oils, 79, 80
  flax seed oil, 79, 80
  linalenic acid, 79, 83
  linoleic acid, 79, 83
  pumpkin seed oil, 79, 80
  soybean oil, 79, 80
  walnut oil, 79, 80
  cis fatty acids, 80
  corn oil, 81
  docosahoxanoic acid, 80
  eicosapentanoic acid, 80
  extra virgin olive oil, 80
  fish oil, 81
  omega-3, 81
  trans fatty acid, 80
Exercise, 115-117
Exercise:
  aerobic exercise, 116
  jogging, 116, 117
  weight training, 116-117
Exercise and fat loss, 26

F

Fat and:
  breast cancer, 30
  colon cancer 30
  prostate cancer, 30
Fat contents of food, 32, 33
Fat contents of snacks, 37, 38, 39
Fat intake and:
  cancer incidence, 30
  fat loss, 25
Fat intake, reducing, 32
Fat loss, 25
Fat loss and:
  chromium, 26
  exercise, 26

Fat Loss and (con't):
  fat intake, 25
  fish oils, 26
  omega-3 fatty acids, 26
Fat loss rules, 25, 26
Fat in American diet, 30
Fat, shopping for 35, 36
Fatty acids, omega-3, 81
Felig, L, 26
Fiber and colorectal cancer, 41
Fiber, 40, 41
  high fiber foods, 43
  intake required, 42
Fish, 93
Fish:
  contaminated, 93
  safe, 93
Fish oils, 81
Fish oils and fat loss, 26
Fisher, Michelle, 22
Five year survival rate, 4
Flax seed oil, 79, 80
Fluorescent light, 108, 109
Food & Drug Administration, 94, 100, 112
Food degradation, 57
Food labels, misleading, 34
Food pollution 88-97
Food pollution at home, 97
Food:
  nitrites in, 64, 65
  organic, 91
  protection, 91, 92
Foran, Jeffrey, 89
Formaldehyde, 99, 100
  in homes, 103, 104

G

Garvin Institute of Medical Research, 26
General Accounting Office (GAO), 2, 4,
Gofman, John, 114
Gorsuch, Anne, 99
Great Lakes, pollution, 93
Greenfield, Ellen, 105

H

Hair spray, 100
Hammer, Armand, 122
Harvard Medical School, 18
Harvard, School of Public Health, 2
Health & Nutrition Examination Survey, 53, 54
High fat foods, 32, 33, 34, 35, 36
High fiber diet, 40
Hoffman, David, 107
Host resistance, 122

I

Immune system, 74
Immune system and antioxidants, 74 - 77
Industrial carcinogens, 98

J

Japanese diet, 30
Jones, Peter, 65

K

Kaiser Health Plan, 118
Knekt, Paul, 69
Kummet, Thomas, 67

L

L-Glutathione, 70

L-Glutathione and:
aging, 70, 71
reduced cancer, 70, 71
LaChance, Paul, 22
Lang, Calvin, 70
Lead in canned food, 97
Lead pollution, 97
Linalenic acid, 79, 83
Linoleic acid, 79, 83
Lipoprotein lipase, 21
Liver cancer, 100
London School of Tropical Medicine, 109
Los Angeles, coastal pollution, 93
Loss of nutrients in food, 58
low fat diet, 30
Low fat foods, 33, 36
Lung cancer, 4, 100
five year survival rate, 5

M

Mammograms, 119-120
Maverick Ranch Beef, 95
McCay, Clive, 27
Mean inspections, 94
Meat, pollutants in, 89
Medawar, Peter, 9
Medical diets, 24
Medication:
cancer causing, 112, 113
diethylstilbestrol, 113
Medifast, 24
Melanoma, 107-109
Melanoma and:
selenium, 69
Metabolism and:
white bread, 49, 50
Methylene chloride, 100
Meyskins, Frank, 67
Minerals - basic formula, 62
Minerals, 53
calcium, 54
chromium, 55
coenzyme Q10, 73
iron, 54
l-glutathione, 70, 71
magnesium, 54
zinc, 55, 111
Minerals, amount required:
selenium, 69
coenzyme Q10, 73
Minerals and reduced cancer:
beta carotene, 67, 68
coenzyme Q10, 73
selenium, 69
Miquel, Jaime, 70
Mitchell, D. 97
Multi-nutrient supplementation, effects on athletic performance, 55
Mushrooms, 96
Mustard, 96
National Cancer Institute (NCI) 1, 11, 15, 17, 28, 40, 42, 50, 53, 63, 119
National Cancer Institute, failure to reduce cancer 2
National Cancer Institute, objection 3
National Gardening Research Center, 106
National Research Council, 17, 30
Nationwide Food Consumption Survey, 54
New England Research Institute, 73
New York Times, 30
Nitrites in food, 64, 65
Nitrosamines, 65
Nixon, Richard 1, 6
Nutrient deficits of US diet, 54, 55, 56
Nutrients:
in soil, 57
loss of in food, 58
Nutrient protection from ultra-violet, 110, 111
Nutrition & Fitness, 2

O

Obesity, 20
Occupational Safety and Health Administration, 100
Oils:
- cold pressed, 79, 80
- cooking, 81, 82, 84
- corn, 81
- flax seed, 79, 80
- olive, extra virgin, 80
- pumpkin seed, 79, 80
- soybean, 79, 80
- walnut, 79, 80
- fish 81

Olive oil, extra virgin, 80
Omega-3 fatty acids, 81
Omega-3 fatty acids and fat loss, 26
Optifast, 24
Oregon Health Sciences University, 21
Overmedication, hazards of, 113
Overweight, 11, 19
Overweight and
- breast cancer, 20
- colorectal cancer, 20
- gall bladder cancer, 20
- ovarian cancer, 20
- prostate cancer, 20
- uterine cancer, 20

Oxybenzone, 110
Ozone Layer, 69, 107
Ozone Treaty, 108

P

Pap Smear, 118
Papanicolaou, George, 118
Para-amino-benzoic acid, 110
Pauling, Linus, 64
Peanut butter, 96
Pesticides:, 11
- benomyl, 90
- chlordineform, 90
- DDT, 89
- deildrin, 89
- dichlorvos, 90
- di ofal, 90
- heptachlor, 89
- mancozeb, 90
- parathon, 89
- phosmet, 90
- trifluralin, 90

Pesticides, to minimize in produce, 92
Peto, Richard, 11
Physician's Desk Reference, 112
Pollutants in meat, 89
Pollution:
- coastal Los Angeles, 93
- food, 88-97
- food, at home, 97
- Great Lakes, 93
- lead, 97
- Puget Sound, 93
- San Francisco Bay, 93

Pollution, testing for water pollutants, 85
Popular diets, 23
Poultry, drug free, 95
Prostaglandin, 81
Prostate cancer & fat, 30
Pumpkin seed oil, 79, 80

R

Radon gas, 103, 104
RDAs, 23, 24, 54, 75
Red wine, 96
Reinhold, V, 69
Reverse osmosis, 86
Richard Simmons Diet, 22
Risk factors, 9
Ross, Maurice, 27, 28

S

San Francisco Bay pollution, 93
Scarsdale Diet, 22
Schroeder, Henry, 58
Selenium, amount required, 69
Selenium and:
  melanoma, 69
  skin damage, 69
  reduced cancer, 69
  skin damage, 69
Sigmoidoscopy, 119
Silverman, J., 30
Simmons, Richard Diet, 22
Skin damage and selenium, 69
Sloan Kettering Hospital, 122
Smith, Eileen, 2
Smoking, 14
Smoking and:
  bladder cancer, 14
  kidney cancer, 15
  lung cancer, 14,
  mouth cancer, 15
  pancreas cancer, 15
  throat cancer, 15
  uterine cancer, 15
Smoking, second hand smoke, 14, 15
Soil, nutrients in 57
Soybean oil, 79, 80
Sputum tests, 120
Squamous cell carcinoma, 107
Steinman, David, 93
Stillman Diet, 22
Stool samples, 119
Storlien, Leonard, 26
Streep, Meryl, 88
Sugar and bodyfat 25
Sulfamethazine, 94
Sunlight, 107-109
Sunscreens, 110, 111
Surgeon General, 14, 113, 120
Swimming pools:
  carcinogens in, 105
  without chlorine, 105

T

Tanning beds, 108
Tanure, R, 81
Tarn Pure, 105
Tea, 96
Tengerdy, Robert, 74
Testicular examination, 120
Thomas, Lewis, 123
Tree Top, 95
Todhunter, John, 99
Toxic wastes, 5
Trans fatty acids, 80
TwinLabs, 60

U

Ultra-violet, 107-109
Ultra-violet, nutrient protection, 110, 111
Underfeeding 27, 28
Uniroyal Chemical, 88
University of Bonn, 69
University of California, 11, 65, 69, 108, 114
University of California:
  Medical School, 27
University of Iowa, 2
University of Louisville, 70
University of Minnesota, 46
University of Southern Africa, 81
University of Southern California, 65
University of Sydney, 109
US diet:
  composition, 57
  nutrient deficits, 54, 55, 56
USDA, 25
UVA, UVB, 108, 109

V

Van de Camp, John, 5, 89
Vegetables, American intake, 46
Vegetables, anticarcinogens in 44, 45, 46, 48
Vegetables, carcinogenic, 96
Vinyl chloride, 100
Vitamins: 53
- basic formula, 61
- composition of supplements, 59, 60
- vitamin A, 54, 111
- vitamin A, betel nut study, 67, 68
- vitamin A, Japanese study, 67
- vitamin B6, 54, 110
- vitamin C, 44
- vitamin C and reduced cancer
- vitamin C, amount required, 65
- vitamin E, 44
- vitamin E and reduced cancer, 66
- vitamin E, amount required, 66

W

Walford, Roy 27, 28
Walnut oil, 79, 80
War against cancer, 1, 3, 6
Water, 84
Water:
- Clean Water Machine, 86
- cleaning water, 85-87
- contamination, 84
- Kodak water cleaning system, 87
- Seagul IV filter, 86
- testing for pollutants, 85
- water filters, 85-87

Wattenberg, Lee 46
Weber, Hans, 70
Weiss, Ted, 2
Whole grains, best 52
Wildlife Federation, 89
Williams, Roger, 50

X

X-rays, 114
X-rays, chest, 120
X-rays, dental, 114
Xienta Institute for Skin Research, 110

Y

Yale University, 26
Your Personal Vitamin Profile, 55